EVALUATION OF THE MARKEY SCHOLARS PROGRAM

Committee for the Evaluation of the
Lucille P. Markey Charitable Trust Programs in Biomedical Sciences

Board on Higher Education and Workforce

Policy and Global Affairs

NATIONAL RESEARCH COUNCIL
OF THE NATIONAL ACADEMIES

THE NATIONAL ACADEMIES PRESS
Washington, DC
www.nap.edu

THE NATIONAL ACADEMIES PRESS   500 Fifth Street, N.W.   Washington, DC 20001

NOTICE: The project that is the subject of this report was approved by the Governing Board of the National Research Council, whose members are drawn from the councils of the National Academy of Sciences, the National Academy of Engineering, and the Institute of Medicine. The members of the committee responsible for the report were chosen for their special competences and with regard for appropriate balance.

This project was supported by Grant No. 98-1 between the Lucille P. Markey Charitable Trust and the National Academy of Sciences. Any opinions, findings, conclusions, or recommendations expressed in this publication are those of the author(s) and do not necessarily reflect the views of the organizations or agencies that provided support for the project.

International Standard Book Number 0-309-10292-8

Additional copies of this report are available from the National Academies Press, 500 Fifth Street, N.W., Lockbox 285, Washington, DC 20055; (800) 624-6242 or (202) 334-3313 (in the Washington metropolitan area); Internet, http://www.nap.edu

THE NATIONAL ACADEMIES
Advisers to the Nation on Science, Engineering, and Medicine

The **National Academy of Sciences** is a private, nonprofit, self-perpetuating society of distinguished scholars engaged in scientific and engineering research, dedicated to the furtherance of science and technology and to their use for the general welfare. Upon the authority of the charter granted to it by the Congress in 1863, the Academy has a mandate that requires it to advise the federal government on scientific and technical matters. Dr. Ralph J. Cicerone is president of the National Academy of Sciences.

The **National Academy of Engineering** was established in 1964, under the charter of the National Academy of Sciences, as a parallel organization of outstanding engineers. It is autonomous in its administration and in the selection of its members, sharing with the National Academy of Sciences the responsibility for advising the federal government. The National Academy of Engineering also sponsors engineering programs aimed at meeting national needs, encourages education and research, and recognizes the superior achievements of engineers. Dr. Wm. A. Wulf is president of the National Academy of Engineering.

The **Institute of Medicine** was established in 1970 by the National Academy of Sciences to secure the services of eminent members of appropriate professions in the examination of policy matters pertaining to the health of the public. The Institute acts under the responsibility given to the National Academy of Sciences by its congressional charter to be an adviser to the federal government and, upon its own initiative, to identify issues of medical care, research, and education. Dr. Harvey V. Fineberg is president of the Institute of Medicine.

The **National Research Council** was organized by the National Academy of Sciences in 1916 to associate the broad community of science and technology with the Academy's purposes of furthering knowledge and advising the federal government. Functioning in accordance with general policies determined by the Academy, the Council has become the principal operating agency of both the National Academy of Sciences and the National Academy of Engineering in providing services to the government, the public, and the scientific and engineering communities. The Council is administered jointly by both Academies and the Institute of Medicine. Dr. Ralph J. Cicerone and Dr. Wm. A. Wulf are chair and vice chair, respectively, of the National Research Council.

www.national-academies.org

Preface

In response to a request by the Lucille P. Markey Charitable Trust, the National Research Council (NRC) of the National Academies, through the Board on Higher Education and Workforce (BHEW), is conducting an evaluation of the Markey Trust's grant programs in the biomedical sciences. During an interval of 15 years, the Markey Trust spent over $500 million on four programs in the basic biomedical sciences that supported the education and research of graduate students, postdoctoral fellows, junior faculty, and senior researchers. This project addresses two questions: "were these funds well spent?" and "what can others in the biomedical and philanthropic communities learn from the programs of the Markey Trust?"

To accomplish these goals, the committee overseeing the project:

- examined the General Organizational Grants program, intended to catalyze new ways to train Ph.D. and M.D. students in translational research;
- convened a conference of Markey Scholars and Visiting Fellows in 2002;
- reviewed the Research Programs Grants, which provided funding to institutions to support the work of senior investigators;
- evaluated the program for Markey Scholars and Visiting Fellows, which supported young biomedical investigators in their early careers; and
- conducted a workshop to investigate methods used to evaluate funding of biomedical science by philanthropic donors.

This is the fifth in a series of reports that document the activities of the Markey Trust. This report examines the Markey Scholars in Biomedical Science and the Markey Visiting Fellows programs, funded by the Markey Trust between 1985 and 1995. The Markey Scholars program funded outstanding biomedical researchers for up to seven years, focusing on the transition from the postdoctorate to junior faculty status. The goal of the program was to ensure maximum productivity, intellectual growth, and independent research among grantees. The Markey Visiting Fellows program provided two years of postdoctoral funding for outstanding young scientists from the United Kingdom and Australia at leading American research institutions. This report examines the career paths and research outcomes of the Markey grantees and, in the case of the Markey Scholars, examines their progress relative to that of a comparison group. The report also details the Scholar selection process and its impact on Scholar outcomes. Finally, the report makes recommendations to other philanthropic funders of biomedical researchers.

Previously published reports in this series detailing the activities of the Markey Trust are (1) *Bridging the Bed-Bench Gap: Contributions of the Markey Trust*, which examined the General Organizational Grants program; (2) *The Markey Scholars Conference Proceedings*, which summarized presentations and abstracts from the 2002 Markey Scholars Conference held as part of the National Academies evaluation; (3) *Funding Biomedical Research Programs: Contributions of the Markey Trust*, which reviewed the Research Program Grants, and (4) *Enhancing Philanthropy's Support of Biomedical Scientists: Proceedings of a Workshop on Evaluation*, which presented a series of papers on evaluation presented at a workshop conducted by the National Academies. All reports are available through the National Academies Press.

This report has been reviewed in draft form by individuals chosen for their diverse perspectives and technical expertise, in accordance with procedures approved by the National Academies' Report Review Committee. The purpose of this independent review is to provide candid and critical comments that will assist the institution in making its published report as sound as possible and to ensure that the report meets institutional standards for objectivity, evidence, and responsiveness to the study charge. The review comments and draft manuscript remain confidential to protect the integrity of the process.

We wish to thank the following individuals for their review of this report: Howard Garrison, Federation of American Societies for Experimental Biology; Paul Klotman, Mount Sinai Medical Center; Michael Leibowitz, UMDNJ-Robert Wood Johnson Medical School; Henry Riecken, University of Pennsylvania; Nancy Street, University of Texas Southwestern Medical Center; and Keith Yamamoto, University of California, San Francisco.

Although the reviewers listed above have provided many constructive comments and suggestions, they were not asked to endorse the conclusions or recommendations, nor did they see the final draft of the report before its release. The review of this report was overseen by Lyle Jones, University of North Carolina at Chapel Hill. Appointed by the National Academies, he was responsible for making certain that an independent examination of this report was carried out in accordance with institutional procedures and that all review comments were carefully considered. Responsibility for the final content of this report rests entirely with the authoring committee and the institution.

The production of this report was the result of planning and oversight for a sustained period of time by the study Committee. I wish to thank Krystyna Isaacs for her outstanding assistance to this report. She interviewed all the Markey Scholars and Visiting Fellows, transcribed and compiled their responses, and contributed to the sections of the report that describe the outcomes of the interviews. George Reinhart, Study Director, ably assisted the committee in this study.

> Lee Sechrest
> *Chair*
> Committee for the Evaluation of the
> Lucille P. Markey Charitable Trust
> Programs in Biomedical Sciences

Contents

Summary   1

1   Introduction   5
    Charge to the Committee, 5
    Markey Grant Programs, 6

2   Markey Awards in Biomedical Sciences   8
    Development of the Scholars Program, 8
    Markey Scholars Selection Process, 10
    Monitoring the Progress of Scholars, 17
    Markey Scholars Conference, 19

3   Evaluation Methodology   21
    Sources of Data, 22
    Response from Scholars and Comparison Group Members, 27

4   Outcomes for the Markey Scholars   30
    Analyses of CVs, CRISP, and Citation Data, 30
    Interviews of Scholars and Top-Ranked and Competitive
      Candidates, 37

5   Lucille P. Markey Visiting Fellows Program   59
    Evaluation of the Visiting Fellows Program, 61
    Interviews with Markey Fellows, 61

6   Conclusions and Recommendations   65

References   71

Appendixes

A   Committee Members Biographical Information   75
B   History of the Markey Trust   78
C   Lucille P. Markey Charitable Trust Programs   83
D   Markey Scholar Awards in Biomedical Sciences   87
E   United Kingdom and Australian Visiting Fellows   102
F   Interview Guides   108

TABLES

2-1   Initial Scholar Stipend and Research Allowance Schedule, 10

2-2   Number and Characteristics of Nominations for Markey Scholar Awards in Biomedical Science, by Year, 12

2-3   Number of Markey Scholar Nominations, by Nomination Outcome and Year, 15

2-4   Percentage of Applicants who were Women at the Stages of the Markey Award Pathway, 17

2-5   Number of Markey Scholars, by Gender and Degree, 17

3-1   Schedule of Markey Scholar and Comparison Group Interviews, 26

3-2   Number of Comparison Group Members, by Level of Contact, 28

4-1   Differences Among Markey Scholars, Top-Ranked, and Competitive Candidates in Academia on Selected Outcome Measures, 31

4-2   Number and Percentage of Markey Scholars and Top-Ranked and Competitive Candidates in Academia by Faculty Rank, 31

4-3   Mean and Median Number of Journal Articles for Markey Scholars, Top-Ranked Candidates, and Competitive Candidates, by Cycle and Overall, 33

4-4   Mean and Median Number of Citations per Individual and Mean Citations per Article for Markey Scholars, Top-Ranked Candidates, and Competitive Candidates, 35

4-5 Differences in Grant Awards Among Markey Scholars, Top-Ranked Candidates, and Competitive Candidates, 36

4-6 Differences in Grant Awards Among Markey Scholars, Top-Ranked Candidates, and Competitive Candidates in Academia, 36

4-7 Percentage Claiming Independence, by Degree and Group, 38

4-8 Percentage Claiming Independence, by Gender and Group, 39

4-9 Percentage Distribution of Reasons for Selecting First Professional Position, by Group, 41

4-10 Number Who Changed Institutions Between the Completion of Training and Commencement of First Faculty Appointment, by Group and Degree, 43

4-11 Number Who Left Academic Bench Science by the Time of Interview, by Group, 44

4-12 Number of Principal Investigators in Academia, by Laboratory Size and Group, 46

4-13 Percentage of Interviewees Engaged in Commercial Interests, by Type of Interest and Group, 47

4-14 Percentage of Interviewees Engaged in Clinical or Translational Research, by Group, 53

FIGURE

C-1 Distribution of Markey Funding Across Programs and Grant Making, 84

Summary

The Lucille P. Markey Charitable Trust was created as a 15-year, limited-term philanthropy in support of basic medical research by the will of Lucille P. Markey who died on July 24, 1982. Mrs. Markey wished that a trust be established "for the purposes of supporting and encouraging basic medical research." The Trustees, who provided governance for the Markey Trust, targeted its programs to specific needs within the biomedical sciences where funding could potentially make a difference. Three primary areas of support emerged over the life of the Trust targeting:

1. Support of young researchers in the biomedical sciences
2. Funding the establishment, reorganization, or expansion of major biomedical research programs or centers led by established investigators
3. Providing training opportunities in translational research for doctoral and medical students.

During the 15 years following its creation, the Lucille P. Markey Charitable Trust spent more than $500 million in these areas.

In response to a request by the Markey Trustees, the National Research Council established a study committee to evaluate the Markey Trust's grant programs. The evaluation project overseen by this committee addresses two general questions: (1) were the Trust's funds well spent? and (2) what can others learn from the programs of the Markey Trust both as an approach to funding biomedical research and as a model of philanthropy?

The Markey Trustees developed an approach to philanthropy they believed would maximize the impact of the Trust's assets on the biomedical sciences. This approach had the following key attributes:

- Distribute all of the assets of the Trust over a limited period of time, allowing more funds to be distributed in a given year and larger awards to be offered;
- Operate with a small core staff, thereby reducing administrative costs and allowing a higher proportion of funds to be awarded to grantees; and
- Provide funds with only a minimum of required reporting, thereby freeing recipients from the burdensome paperwork often associated with grants.

The Markey Scholar Awards in Biomedical Science and the United Kingdom and Australian Visiting Fellows[1] were developed in response the Trustees' perceived need for funding to enhance the transition from postdoctoral fellow to faculty status. With guidance from expert consultants, the Trustees formulated a program that made about 16 Markey Scholar awards per year to outstanding young biomedical scientists for the seven years between 1985 and 1991 for a total of 113 awards. The program had a rigorous selection process that contributed to its success. The Trustees stipulated that half of the Scholar awardees should have Ph.D. degrees and half should have M.D. or M.D./Ph.D. degrees. The program funded up to 3 years as a postdoctoral fellow followed by 5 years as a faculty member. Stipend and laboratory expenses were included in the funding package that ranged from $570,000 to over $700,000 for Scholars who remained in the program. In addition, between 1986 and 1993 the Trustees supported 36 outstanding young scientists from the United Kingdom and Australia for two-year fellowships at American research institutions.

This report assesses the impact of the Markey Scholars program from three perspectives—were Markey funds well spent, did the Scholars do well, and are there lessons for other funders of biomedical researchers to be gleaned from the Markey Scholars program? The committee adopted a multifaceted approach to evaluating the Markey Scholars program that drew on:

---

[1]The official names of the programs are the Markey Scholar Award in Biomedical Science and the United Kingdom and Australian Visiting Fellows. The terms Scholars Award or Markey Scholars program and Visiting Fellows program will be used throughout the report.

- Resume analysis
- Citation analysis
- Analysis of NIH databases
- Analysis of Markey Trust archival information
- Interviews with Markey Scholars and Visiting Fellows

In order to better understand the career outcomes of the Markey Scholars, the study committee compared indicators of achievement for the Scholars with those for individuals who were unsuccessful applicants for Markey Scholar awards. The Markey Scholars authored more articles, had a higher level of citations per individual and article, received more R01 grants, achieved higher rank, had a shorter time to tenure, and were located in higher ranked institutions than the biomedical scientists in the comparison groups. There was no difference, however, between Scholars and comparison group members in total number of NIH grants.

With only two years of postdoctoral funding, the Visiting Fellows program did not have the same impact as the Markey Scholars program. Nevertheless, it was an invaluable experience for the Visiting Fellows that enriched their research.

Thus, the committee concluded that both the Markey Scholars and Visiting Fellows programs were successful. The committee recognized that there were two aspects of the Markey award that could account for differences between the Markey Scholars and the comparison groups—the process used to select Markey Scholars and the size, structure, and duration of the award itself. The committee concluded that it was unable to differentiate the impacts of these two factors, but that they could evaluate the Markey award program generally.

The committee recommends the following based on its findings:

Recommendation 1. Other funders, especially NIH, should consider creating awards that facilitate the transition from postdoctoral fellow to faculty status. The committee recognizes that the transition from postdoctoral fellow to faculty status can be stressful. Moreover, very few funding programs provide career transition awards, although there has been recognition for their need for such programs for several years.

Recommendation 2. Other funders of biomedical researchers should consider adopting the Markey Scholars Award as a template that can be used by philanthropic and governmental funders (especially the NIH) to identify and fund biomedical scientists at this important time in their careers. The committee recommends that any future funders of career transitions awards give careful consideration to this template since it can enable funders to (1) identify postdoctoral fellows who believe that they are independent or nearly independent in their research agenda, (2) provide funding not only for salaries but also for laboratory equipment, supplies, and staff, and (3) monitor awardees to ensure that they establish independent research careers in a timely manner. The committee urges funders to make certain that institutions making nominations ensure that female and minority nominees are fully included in all aspects of the nomination process. The committee recommends that future funders incorporate annual meetings modeled after the Markey Scholars Conference to enable awardees to benefit from networking. Finally, both the Scholars and comparison group members offered innovative suggestions for features that went beyond the Markey template and might enhance the funding of biomedical scientists. The committee recommends that any future funders consider these suggestions as part of the funding process.

Recommendation 3. The committee recommends funding to foster the international exchange of biomedical scientists for research and training. The committee recommends that funders establish mechanisms to bring foreign biomedical scientists to laboratories in the United States for intensive research and training and to fund research and training opportunities for U.S. biomedical scientists abroad.

Recommendation 4. Any funders of biomedical researchers should incorporate a prospective, data-driven monitoring and evaluation system as part of the program. The committee strongly believes that a data-driven, prospective evaluation should be fully integrated into any new funding initiative. The committee recommends that funders undertake (at least) annual monitoring of awardees activities for several years. Data generated from monitoring should be used to target appropriate candidates and tailor funding to meet changing needs.

Recommendation 5. The biotechnology industry and the government are making important contributions to the biomedical research agenda and should not be excluded from transitional funding mechanisms. The committee recognizes that the biotechnology industry and government are increasingly attractive destinations for biomedical researchers. It recommends current and future funders of biomedical scientists continue support for those who transition to these destinations outside of academia.

I

Introduction

CHARGE TO THE COMMITTEE

During an interval of 15 years, the Lucille P. Markey Charitable Trust[1] spent more than $500 million on three grant programs in the basic biomedical sciences that supported the education and research of graduate students, postdoctoral fellows, junior faculty, and senior researchers. In response to a request from the Markey Trust, the National Research Council (NRC) appointed a study committee to conduct an evaluation of the Trust's grant programs in which it would address two general questions: (1) Were these funds well spent, and (2) What can others in the biomedical and philanthropic communities learn from the programs of the Markey Trust.

To accomplish these goals, the committee[2] overseeing the project:

- examined the General Organizational Grants, intended to catalyze new ways to train Ph.D. and M.D. students in translational research;
- convened a conference of Markey Scholars and Visiting Fellows in 2002;

---

[1]The Lucille P. Markey Charitable Trust is the institution's official name. In this report it will be referred to as the "Markey Trust" or the "Trust."

[2]The Committee for the Evaluation of the Lucille P. Markey Charitable Trust Programs in Biomedical Sciences is the official name of the NRC study committee that will assess the Markey Trust's activities. Hereafter it will be referred to as the committee or the Markey committee.

- assessed the Research Programs Grants, which provided funding to institutions to support the work of senior investigators;
- conducted a workshop to investigate methods used to evaluate funding of biomedical sciences by philanthropic donors; and
- evaluated the program for Markey Scholars and Visiting Fellows, which supported young biomedical investigators in their early careers.

This report presents the findings and conclusions of the evaluation of the Markey Scholars and Visiting fellows programs.

MARKEY GRANT PROGRAMS

The Markey Trust established three programs to support basic training, the development of young faculty, and research by experienced scientists in the biomedical sciences: (1) General Organizational Grants, (2) Research Program Grants; and (3) Markey Scholars and Visiting Fellows Awards. In addition, the Trust awarded several grants that did not fall neatly into one of these categories. For purposes of this evaluation purposes, however, these were assigned to one or another of the programs. A detailed description of all Markey grant programs is included in Appendix C.

General Organizational Grants

The growth of a gap between the results of biomedical research and their clinical application was recognized by Markey trustees as a critical issue in the late 1980s. Consequently, the Markey Trust funded awards to provide training in translational research to diminish this gap, including: (1) programs that provided significant opportunities for M.D.s to engage in basic research during and immediately following medical school and residency, and (2) programs that provided significant clinical exposure for Ph.D.s while they were predoctoral or postdoctoral students. General Organizational Grant programs were funded for approximately five years and were not renewable.

Research Program Grants

The Trust established Research Program Grants to enable established investigators to address important issues in the biomedical sciences by developing new approaches or expanding continuing approaches to the study of basic biomedical research questions—in short, providing flexible dollars for innovation and growth. In some instances, the awards permitted the development of new programs or the complete reorganization of existing programs. In other cases, the awards enhanced existing programs and research endeavors.

Markey Scholars and Visiting Fellows Awards

The Trust also adopted several mechanisms to fund selected scholars early in their careers. The two most important were (1) the Markey Scholar Awards in Biomedical Sciences through which a total of 113 Markey Scholars were supported for up to three years of postdoctoral training followed by five years of support as a junior faculty member with both salary and research funding provided, and (2) the United Kingdom and Australian Visiting Fellows Awards, which funded outstanding young scientists from the United Kingdom and Australia as postdoctoral fellows at American research institutions for two years.

2

Markey Scholar Awards in Biomedical Sciences

DEVELOPMENT OF THE SCHOLARS PROGRAM

Early in its existence, the Markey Trustees recognized the importance of providing funding to promising young biomedical scientists at the point of launching their careers. In April 1984, the Trust convened a one-day meeting of distinguished experts in the biomedical sciences to consider the ways in which the Trust could contribute to the biomedical research community. Many important ideas emerged from this meeting in Palo Alto, California, some of which subsequently evolved into Markey funded programs. One theme that was emphasized throughout the meeting was the need to support promising young investigators, especially as biomedical research fellowship funding had not kept pace with the needs of researchers seeking to transition from postdoctoral positions to independent research careers. The Trust conducted a second meeting of experts in the biomedical sciences in New York City in May, 1984. Many of the ideas for funding targets that surfaced during the meeting in Palo Alto were echoed in the New York meeting. From these two meetings, the framework of a mechanism to fund promising young biomedical scientists began to take shape.

The experts were concerned that the number of NIH-supported postdoctoral trainees and new awards to young scientists had been decreasing (National Institutes of Health, 2001, 2003), as was postdoctoral support from other funders such as the American Cancer Society. In addition, the group recognized that the funding level of most postdoctoral fellowships was too low to support physicians or scientists 7 or 8 years beyond their baccalaureate. Moreover, there was a consensus that M.D.s were at a competitive disadvantage with Ph.D. scientists for postdoctoral fellowships. Finally, the experts pointed out that the move from postdoctoral fellow to junior faculty was a difficult transition. The development of a career in independent research required that junior faculty devote considerable time and effort to research with salary and research support assured. Yet NIH funding mechanisms were not designed to foster the independent research careers of new faculty. The long lead time required, the difficulty in developing independent pilot data, and the complexity of the NIH review process, combined with the limited funding available worked against the development of an independent research career for young scientists.

As a result of the deliberations that occurred at the two meetings, the Trust crafted a program to fund young scientists with the potential to contribute significantly to biomedical research. This program, the Markey Scholars Awards program, was a hybrid funding mechanism that combined postdoctoral training with the first faculty appointment. Scholars Awards provided adequate support for both the postdoctoral period as well as for the initial years of the faculty appointment, to maximize productivity, foster intellectual growth, and encourage independence. Under the conditions of the Trust, a total of 16 Markey Scholar Awards were to be made each year, half to applicants with Ph.D. degrees and half to applicants with either M.D. or M.D./Ph.D. degrees.

The Trustees recognized the special circumstances of some M.D. and M.D./Ph.D. scientists who are required to spend up to 3 years of clinical residency training. Such individuals require an additional 3 or 4 years of postdoctoral support, before obtaining a faculty position in a clinical or basic sciences department. By contrast, the Ph.D.s will have completed their postdoctoral fellowship and will be ready to assume faculty status at a much earlier point in their career. Recognizing these different career pathways, the Trustees determined that Ph.D. scientists would be eligible for nomination at the start of their second or third year postdoctoral year and would receive funding for an additional two years of the postdoctorate and that M.D.s and M.D./Ph.D.s would be eligible for nomination at the start of their last year of clinical training or after 1 year of postdoctoral training and they included funding for 3 years of postdoctoral training. All nominees were eligible for 5 years of funding at the faculty level.

In addition, the Trustees concluded that it was appropriate to fund a research allowance (varying from $15,000 to $60,000) for all Scholars. The research allowance was modest during the postdoctoral years; increased substantially during the initial faculty years; and was reduced during the final faculty years in anticipation of other extramural funding. Finally, recognizing the potential for additional education debt for Scholars with

TABLE 2-1 Initial Scholar Stipend and Research Allowance Schedule

	Basic Science Ph.D.		M.D. and M.D./Ph.D.	
Year of Award	Stipend	Research Allowance	Stipend	Research Allowance
Postdoctoral Year 1	N/A	N/A	$30,000	$15,000
Postdoctoral Year 2	N/A	N/A	$33,000	$15,000
Postdoctoral Year 3	$25,000	$15,000	$36,000	$15,000
Postdoctoral Year 4	$28,000	$15,000	N/A	N/A
Faculty Year 1	$35,000	$60,000	$45,000	$60,000
Faculty Year 2	$40,000	$50,000	$50,000	$50,000
Faculty Year 3	$45,000	$50,000	$55,000	$50,000
Faculty Year 4	$50,000	$25,000	$60,000	$25,000
Faculty Year 5	$55,000	$15,000	$65,000	$15,000
Total	$280,000	$225,000	$380,000	$245,000

SOURCE: Lucille P. Markey Scholar Awards in Biomedical Science, 1984.

a M.D. or M.D./Ph.D. degree, their additional years of training, and their need for more postdoctoral training the Trustees concluded that it would be appropriate to offer them higher stipends than for Scholars with a Ph.D. degree. The initial stipend and research allowance schedule is shown in Table 2-1.

In 1988, the Trustees increased the starting level of postdoctoral and faculty stipends for Markey Scholars by $5000. At the same time, the Trustees modified the policy on postdoctoral fellowships, enabling some Scholars to continue their postdoctoral fellowships for an additional year. Actual Scholar awards ranged from $570,000 to $711,000 depending on the length of the postdoctoral experience and the Scholar's degree. The Markey Trust was unique in providing support for young scientists for up to 8 years, committing a total funding of $59,795,900 for the Markey Scholars program.

MARKEY SCHOLARS SELECTION PROCESS

During the 7 years of the Scholars Awards program, the total number of nominations for Awards was 1,212. Individuals could be and, in some cases were, nominated more than once, so the number of individuals nominated for the Markey Scholars Awards program was 1,154. The nomination process began with a formal, written request for nominations from deans of medical schools, senior administrative officials of selected research universities without medical schools, and from research institutes with a strong interest in biomedical science. Moreover, beginning in 1987, the Trust placed notices in *Science*, *Nature*, the *New England Journal of Medicine*, and the *Journal of Clinical Investigation* describing the Markey Award and the application process. The request for nominations outlined the conditions of the award:

- Scholars were to devote no less than 90 percent of their time to research.
- Scholars could receive salary supplements from other sources without prior approval from the Trust.
- Scholars were required to submit annual budgets.
- Approval of the Selection Committee was required for equipment purchases in excess of $2000.
- Scholars were required to submit annual progress reports.
- Scholars could relocate to other institutions with the expectation that the move would enhance academic and research growth, but prior approval of the Selection Committee was required.
- Scholars were expected to conform to the host institution's regulations on the use of humans and vertebrate animals in research.
- Scholars were expected to share research findings through recognized publications and presentations at scientific forums.

As can be seen from the data reported in Table 2-2, consistency in the nominations was remarkable over the years with respect to number of nominations, sex of nominees, and M.D. vs. Ph.D. status. Not surprisingly, the maximum number of nominations occurred in the first year of the program. One important trend in the program, however, was the decrease in the number of institutions submitting nominations: from 100 during the initial funding cycle to about 64 during the last four funding cycles. That decrease may reflect the quality of Scholars selected during the initial funding cycles, the complexity of the application package, and the rigor of the Scholar selection process. It may be that some universities whose candidates were not selected may have stopped submitting nominations. Moreover, the decline in the number of institutions submitting the maximum number of nominations also decreased substantially over the course of the program. That change may be due to the increase from 4 to 6 in the number of nominations allowed.

Nomination packages, consisting of the following eight components, were received by the Trust's administrative office by mid-November of the year preceding the award:

1. A letter from the faculty sponsor detailing the nominee's qualifications and research environment.

TABLE 2-2 Number and Characteristics of Nominations for Markey Scholar Award in Biomedical Science, by Year

Nominations for Scholar Awards in Biomedical Science	Year							Total
	1985	1986	1987	1988	1989	1990	1991	
Number of Nominations	216	184	178	126	145	186	177	1,212
Number (Percent) Female	34 (17)	38 (21)	46 (26)	35 (28)	34 (23)	52 (28)	40 (22)	270 (23)
Number (Percent) Ph.D.s	129 (60)	112 (61)	103 (58)	78 (62)	84 (58)	113 (61)	111 (63)	730 (60)
Number of Institutions Submitting Nominations	100	75	77	64	62	65	66	—
Number of Institutions with Maximum Nominations[a]	17	4	6	2	4	4	5	—

[a]In 1985 institutions could make up to 4 nominations, thereafter 6 nominations was the maximum.
SOURCE: Lucille P. Markey Charitable Trust Records.

2. A letter of endorsement from the head of department or research unit.

3. A letter of endorsement from the senior academic officer.

4. A copy of the nominee's full curriculum vitae.

5. A complete bibliography.

6. A letter of support from the dissertation advisor or chief of service.

7. Letters of recommendation from additional faculty who knew the nominee's current research well.

8. A statement outlining a plan for research over the period of the award along with long-term career objectives. This statement was limited to 10 double-spaced typewritten pages, half of which was devoted to the research plan and half to research following completion of the fellowship.

When institutions submitted their nomination packages, the Markey administration office recorded its arrival, checked it for eligibility and completeness, and sent copies of the nomination package to the chairman and vice-chairman of the selection committee (Box 2-1) for initial screening. The chairman and vice-chairman reviewed all nominees and, if they agreed that an application was not competitive, they classified it as unsuccessful. In cases in which there was a split decision, additional selection committee members were consulted. Competitive nominations received a second review by the selection committee (see Table 2-3). A total of 1,212 nomination packages were received over the seven-year period. Out of these, 83 were incomplete or ineligible. Of the rest, the chairman and vice-chairman of the selection committee deemed 605 unsuccessful and 524 (43 percent of all nominations) competitive and worthy to be reviewed by the entire selection committee.

In the second phase of the selection process, each member of the selection committee was sent successful nomination packages for review, usually between 12 and 15 so that two selection committee members reviewed each nominee. The chairman made sure that no selection committee member reviewed a nominee who had an institutional affiliation the same as the selection committee member. One member of the selection committee was assigned as the primary reviewer and the other as the secondary reviewer. Each selection committee member was asked to list the four highest ranking nominees and then send the ranked listing to the chairman of the selection committee.

The chairman of the Selection Committee compiled all the listings of top-ranked candidates. There were ten members of the selection committee; each submitted four candidates; so the maximum potential was 40 top-ranked candidates. These were forwarded to the Trust's administrative office. The administrative office distributed the compiled listing to the entire selection committee for consideration at the Scholar Selection Committee meeting. The two assigned reviewers brought one-page reviews of the applicant, the proposed research, and the institutional environment, and made oral presentations to the selection committee. Following presentations on all applicants and a thorough discussion, committee members voted by written ballot, assigning priority scores from 1 to 5 as in a NIH study section. Awards were assigned on the basis of the aggregated priority scores. The differences in the priority scores between those who became Scholars and the rest of the top-ranked candidates were very small. Anecdotal evidence shows that the Selection Committee thought of the Scholars and top-ranked candidates who were not selected as "peas in a pod" (Lucille P. Markey Charitable Trust Records). However, the Scholar Selection Committee was restricted in the number of Scholars that could be appointed each year.

As shown in Table 2-3, over the seven-years of the program, there were 115 Scholar Awards, 186 top-ranked candidates who did not receive

BOX 2-1
Scholar Selection Committee

The initial Scholar Selection Committee, formed in 1984, consisted of the following 10 distinguished biomedical scientists:

Purnell W. Choppin, M.D., Chairman
Vice President for Academic Programs and Leon Hess Professor of Virology
The Rockefeller University

David M. Kipnis, M.D., Vice Chairman
Busch Professor and Chairman, Department of Medicine
Washington University School of Medicine

Bruce M. Alberts, Ph.D.
American Cancer Society Lifetime Research Professor
Professor, Department of Biochemistry and Biophysics
University of California, San Francisco

Alfred G. Gilman, M.D., Ph.D.
Professor and Chairman, Department of Pharmacology
University of Texas Southwestern Medical School

Leroy E. Hood, M.D., Ph.D.
Chairman of the Division of Biology
California Institute of Technology

Roger D. Kornberg, Ph.D.
Professor and Chairman, Department of Cell Biology
Stanford University School of Medicine

Philip Leder, M.D.
Chairman, Department of Genetics
Harvard Medical School

Thomas D. Pollard, M.D.
Chairman, Department of Cell Biology & Anatomy
The Johns Hopkins University School of Medicine

Janet D. Rowley, M.D.
Professor of Medicine
University of Chicago Pritzker School of Medicine

Charles F. Stevens, M.D., Ph.D.
Professor and Chairman, Section of Molecular Neurobiology
Yale University School of Medicine

continued

BOX 2-1 Continued

In 1985, Dr. Choppin became president of the Howard Hughes Medical Institute (HHMI) and resigned his position on the selection committee. Dr. Kipnis assumed the position of chairman and Dr. Leder assumed the position of vice-chairman. The vacant position on the selection committee was filled by:

Malcolm A. Martin, M.D.
Chief, Laboratory of Molecular Microbiology
National Institute of Allergy and Infectious Diseases, NIH

In 1987, Drs. Kornberg and Rowley resigned from the selection committee. Their positions were filled by:

John A. Oates, M.D.
Professor and Chairman, Department of Medicine
Vanderbilt University

Shirley M. Tilghman, Ph.D.
Professor of Molecular Biology
Princeton University

TABLE 2-3 Number of Markey Scholar Nominations, by Nomination Outcome and Year

| | Nomination Outcomes | | | | |
Year	Individuals Receiving Scholar Award	Top-Ranked Candidates Not Receiving Scholar Award	Other Competitive Candidates Not Top-Ranked	Ineligible, Incomplete, or Unsuccessful	Total
1985	16	18	47	135	216
1986	16	23	34	111	184
1987	16	27	28	107	178
1988	17	27	30	52	126
1989	17	29	33	66	145
1990	17	31	27	111	186
1991	15	31	24	106	177
Total	115	186	223	688	1,212

SOURCE: Lucille P. Markey Charitable Trust Records.

awards, 223 others who were considered competitive but who were not top-ranked, and 688 whose applications were considered unsuccessful (did not pass the first screening). Individuals were eligible to be nominated more than once; in fact, 58 persons were nominated two times. For Scholars, top-ranked candidates, other competitive candidates, and not reviewed nominees, the number of duplicate nominations was 9, 14, 14, and 21 respectively. Consequently, the total numbers of nominees in the four categories were actually 115, 177, 209, and 653 respectively. Since 83 application packages were either ineligible or incomplete and, consequently, were never considered for an award, the total number of nominees considered for the Scholars Award in Biomedical Sciences was 1,071.

The selection committee was frequently faced with a surfeit of riches, especially of applicants with Ph.D. degrees who were highly qualified for the Scholar award. However, the annual awards were meant to be divided equally between Ph.D.s, on the one hand, and M.D. or M.D./Ph.D.s, on the other. So, the selection committee ranked all Ph.D. candidates in one column and all M.D.s and M.D./Ph.D.s in another, and then selected the top individuals, targeting half of the awards to each group. Because of the constraints imposed by the Trust, the selection committee was in the unenviable position of making Markey Scholar Awards to M.D.s or M.D./Ph.D.s with lower priority scores than some of the highly rated Ph.D. applicants. Moreover, because 60 percent of applicants were Ph.D.s, the probability of a given Ph.D. receiving an award—.08—was 50 percent lower than the probability of an individual M.D. or M.D./Ph.D. receiving an award—.12.

The selection committee's concerns about the outcomes of physician Scholars relative to and scientist Scholars, however, were not borne out in reality. The results of the analyses of resumes, CRISP, and citation analysis show that the differences between scientist and physician Scholars were small. In fact, for scholarly productivity (journal articles) and the total number of NIH grants, physician scholars had better outcomes that did Scholars with Ph.D. degrees.

A second area of concern to the Markey Trustees was the percentage of Markey Scholar awards given to women (Markey Archival Data). At the conclusion of the initial awards (the class of 1985), the Trustees began monitoring the gender of applicants at the various stages of the award pathway (see Table 2-4). Variations in the percentage of Markey Scholars Awards made to women result from the very small number involved. The committee is aware that the data collected for the outcome measures used in this study may have been affected by both the low response rates of persons in the two comparison groups and the lower than expected number of females among Markey Scholar candidates. The latter factor,

TABLE 2-4 Percentage of Applicants Who Were Women at the Stages of the Markey Award Pathway

Stages of Markey Award Pathway	Cycle							Total
	1	2	3	4	5	6	7	
Markey Scholars	18.8	12.5	31.3	23.5	11.8	17.6	18.8	19.5
Top-Ranked	16.7	26.1	29.6	25.9	17.2	16.1	3.2	18.8
Competitive	12.8	20.6	14.3	30.0	24.2	22.2	8.3	18.8
Unsuccessful	18.5	24.3	28.0	30.8	31.8	31.5	32.1	27.3
Total Applicants	17.1	22.8	26.4	28.6	24.8	26.3	22.6	23.7

SOURCE: Lucille P. Markey Charitable Trust Records.

however, would not have influenced the analytical comparisons since the percent of Markey Scholars who are women (19.5%) is similar to the percent of women in each of the two comparison groups (18.8%), as shown in Table 2-4.

A total of 115 Markey Scholar Awards were offered to worthy candidates. Two awardees declined to accept their awards as they had also been offered positions as HHMI Investigators. Unable to accept both awards, they selected the HHMI award. The distribution of Markey Scholars by gender and degree is shown in Table 2-5. Awards were made to 91 male (80 percent) and 22 female (20 percent) scientists. Half of the awardees (n = 57) had Ph.D. degrees and half (n = 56) had M.D. or M.D./Ph.D. degrees.

TABLE 2-5 Number of Markey Scholars, by Gender and Degree

Gender	Degree			Total
	M.D.	M.D./Ph.D.	Ph.D.	
Male	17	30	44	91
Female	2	7	13	22
Total	19	37	57	113

MONITORING THE PROGRESS OF SCHOLARS

The Scholars Selection Committee served not only to screen and select Scholars, but also to monitor their progress while they were receiving Markey funding and to ensure that they were making progress toward the goals of productivity and independence. Scholars were required to submit annual progress reports along with financial reports from their host institution. The selection committee reviewed these progress reports annually. The selection committee was especially concerned with Scholars' progress at two important points in their career pathway: the transition from postdoctoral fellow to faculty status, and the midpoint of their Markey faculty funding. These annual reports and reviews by the selection committee were critical milestones for Scholars. Subsequent year funding was not authorized until a complete annual report was received and approved. Moreover, funds could also be held up at the times of selection committee reviews if scholarship and progress toward independence was not demonstrated. For two Scholars, funding was terminated before the completion of the award tenure.

As Scholars made the transition from postdoctoral fellow to assistant professor, the Scholar's primary and secondary reviewers scrutinized the new appointment from two perspectives. First, the reviewers wanted to ensure that the new appointment would contribute to establishing an independent research agenda for the Scholar. Second, they wanted to ensure that the host institution would comply with the Markey Trust's stipulations for Scholars—90 percent time devoted to research, adequate laboratory space and start-up package, and enhancement of academic and research growth.

Approximately two years later, as Scholars entered into the third (of five) years of funding at the faculty level, they received a second review from their primary and secondary reviewers. Here the selection committee reviewers were focusing on the Scholars' progression toward research independence. The reviewers were particularly concerned with productivity and grant activity (Lucille P. Markey Charitable Trust Records). A sample of comments from the Scholars Selection Committee gives examples of their concern. In most cases, the comments were brief and positive, but in some showed the concern of the members of the Scholar Selection Committee.

> *[Scholar] is approved through the third faculty year with the award ending in 6/30/92 and is eligible for two additional years.*

> *The following Class V Scholars are approved for support through their fifth faculty year (a list of 13 Scholars is attached).*

> *I am concerned that [Scholar] still continues to publish primarily as a member of a group with only one senior authored paper in a review journal. To participate as a member of a group is fine but by the time [the Scholar] is entering the third year of faculty appointment there should be more evidence of independence and leadership.*

This is an ambitious project that also carries an element of risk, as reflected by the lack of any mention of publications. It deserves careful scrutiny. A phone call to assess whether the lack of mentioned publications is an oversight or a real reflection of the publication record would seem in order. This candidate should be reviewed at the Scholars Conference before any decision to move to faculty appointment.

[Scholar's] research progress was discussed at length and it was decided that [Reviewer] would meet with [Scholar] to express the committee's concerns. They will also offer suggestions for enhancing research training. [Scholar] was approved for funding for one additional year only, with special progress reviews scheduled biannually. [Scholar] will be advised following the last review if the Scholar Award will be extended.

This Scholar continues to worry me. In faculty year 3, he still has not applied for competitive research funds from a national source. The work seems to be solid, but somewhat obscure. Nevertheless, I have no strong reasons to discontinue support.

The Selection Committee had the authority to terminate the award for Scholars who did not meet expectations of research productivity or independence. In a few cases, Scholars received tersely written warnings that funding would be ended unless and until the Selection Committee was satisfied with the Scholar's demonstration of progress and independence

Scholars who left academia for the pharmaceutical or biotechnology industry were required to forego their Markey awards; four Scholars left for attractive opportunities in industry. Ten Scholars elected to accept HHMI investigatorships and, consequently, resigned their Markey awards. One Scholar was recruited by NIH and two Scholars accepted positions overseas—one at the European Molecular Biology Organization and one returned to his home country (Japan). Finally, two Scholars were terminated for failure to demonstrate progress in their research agendas and make satisfactory progress toward independence. All Markey Scholars were included in this study, including those who were terminated and those who were required to relinquish their Markey support to accept HHMI investigatorships or accept positions outside of academia.

MARKEY SCHOLARS CONFERENCE

One of the important features of the Markey award was the annual Scholars Conference. The conference was conducted annually from 1986 until 1996, usually during the month of September. In addition to Markey Scholars and Visiting Fellows, attendees included members of the Scholars

Selection Committee, Markey Trustees, and invited guests. Initially, all Scholars and Visiting Fellows presented posters, but as the number attending the conference increased, posters were presented by a sample of Scholars and Fellows with the rest submitting abstracts. Conferences featured keynote presentations by established biomedical researchers. Some conferences were themed: the 1995 Scholar's Conference, for example, presented a symposium on clinical research in molecular medicine.

Scholars reported that the conference was an important opportunity to network, not only with other Scholars, but also with the members of the Scholar Selection Committee and with the invited guests. In addition, the Selection Committee members used the conference as an opportunity to meet with Scholars and mentor them. The Scholars volunteered that they welcomed and valued guidance from the Selection Committee members. Scholars, who had relinquished their Scholar award, either because they left academic research for the biotechnology industry or accepted a HHMI investigatorship, were not invited to attend the subsequent Scholars' Conferences. When interviewed, these Scholars stated that the thing that they regretted most was not being able to attend the Scholars' Conference.

3

Evaluation Methodology

The committee was asked to assess whether the Markey Trust's funds were well spent and what others could learn from the programs of the Markey Trust both as an approach to funding biomedical research and as a model of philanthropy. For purposes of this report, the committee was particularly interested in determining if there was evidence that the Markey Scholar award gave a particular and singular advantage to Scholars that enabled them to reach scientific independence, career progression, and positions of leadership in the scientific community earlier than a similar group of postdoctoral fellows without the Markey award. The committee recognized that there were two aspects of the Markey award that could account for differences between the Markey Scholars and a comparable group of postdoctoral fellows. One was the process used to select Markey Scholars, a process designed to ensure that only outstanding researchers were selected. The other was the size, structure, and duration of the award itself. The committee concluded that it was unable to differentiate the impacts of these two factors, and that they could only evaluate the Markey award program generally.

To do this, the committee identified measures that would indicate scientific independence, research productivity and professional success, and selected the following five as particularly salient:

1. Appointment to a tenure-track position in a top-ranked Research I university
2. Promotion and tenure to associate and full professor
3. Publishing rate

4. Citations per individual and per article

5. Success in achieving extramural funding, especially a traditional NIH research program award (R01)

In addition, the committee determined that the use of a comparison group would strengthen its ability to assess the relative impact of the Markey award on the Scholars' outcomes. The committee established three criteria to use in searching for possible comparison groups for the evaluation of the Markey Scholars. First, they specifically sought programs that provided transitional funding for postdocs, not funding to faculty (persons with faculty status were ineligible for the Markey Scholar award). Second, they sought programs that provided initial funding for approximately the same time as the Markey Scholars, 1985 through 1991. Finally, they sought programs that provided generous funding for seven years that included both stipend/salary funding as well as funds for laboratory expenses. The committee could find no programs that met these criteria. The NIH K22 awards did not begin until 1998. The Burroughs Wellcome awards, based on the Markey award, did not begin until 1995. The American Heart Association fellow-to-faculty awards did not begin until 2002. Career development awards made by Pew, Searle, American Cancer Society, American Heart Association, Sloan, Keck, and Beckman are all oriented toward funding faculty and generally speaking provide funding for only 3 or 4 years. Markle awards were restricted to physicians.

The committee concluded that the best comparison group would be candidates who were considered for the Markey Award but who did not receive it. After examining the Scholar selection process, the committee decided that two comparison groups could be identified. The first comparison group was composed of candidates who were top-ranked but not selected (referred to in this report as "top-ranked candidates"). The second comparison group consisted of candidates who were competitive, but not top-ranked (referred to in this report as "competitive candidates").

SOURCES OF DATA

The evaluation of the Markey Scholars Program presented the committee with some interesting considerations. First, the outcome of the evaluation would not inform the Markey Trust, which no longer existed. Rather the evaluation would inform others in the philanthropic community that supported the training and research of biomedical scientists. Second, whatever approach to evaluation the committee selected, the approach would be a hybrid: a combination of both a prospective and a retrospective assessment.

All, or nearly all, of the Markey Scholars had completed their awards by the time of the initial meeting of the National Academies committee in 1998. However, the Markey Trustees realized that any evaluation of the Scholars program would require data collection well beyond the end of the Markey Trust. They envisioned an evaluation that would be completed in 2007 (Lucille P. Markey Charitable Trust Records) and commissioned the National Research Council of the National Academies to conduct a prospective evaluation that would culminate about 10 years after the Trust ceased operation.

The committee identified five sources of information that would inform its evaluation of the Markey Scholars. Three sources provided quantitative data:

1. Curriculum vitae of Markey Scholars and comparison group members
2. Citations of articles published by Markey Scholars and comparison group members
3. Data on extramural funding of Markey Scholars and comparison group members

Two additional sources provided qualitative information:

4. Data collected by the Markey Trust
5. Interviews with Scholars and comparison group members.

Quantitative Data

Curriculum vitae (CV) submitted by Scholars and comparison group members at the time of their interview. All Scholars and comparison group members were asked to submit a complete CV at the time of their interview. The CV analysis was used to extract data on career progress such as rank, tenure, promotions, honors and awards. It was also used to extract data on productivity such as licenses, patents, and journal articles.

For the publication analysis, counts were made of journal articles listed on an individual's CV for a 14-year period beginning with the year in which the individual received or would have received the Markey Scholar Award. The 14-year range was chosen because it was assumed that all individuals in the study would have achieved their first professional position (i.e., became faculty members if they stayed in academia) within 4 years and the evaluation sought to follow up 10 years later. Consequently, all Scholars, top-ranked, and competitive candidates were compared over an interval of the same length.

Data on citations. While journal articles provide an indicator of productivity, citations for these articles provide a measure of overall scholarly impact. The number of citations for journal articles written by Scholars and comparison group members were obtained from the Institute for Scientific Information (ISI). NRC staff submitted permutations of the names of all Scholars and comparison group members in ISI format (e.g., J Smith and JB Smith for John B. Smith), indicating the years of interest for the biological and biomedical sciences broadly defined. Using current CVs for Scholars and for both candidate groups, NRC staff linked journal articles from the CV for the 14-year period used in counting publications (see above and Figure 3-1) to the ISI citation database which provided citations for these articles for the period through 2004. So, for example, using articles published by Scholars and comparison group members in cycle 1 for the period 1985-1998, we counted citations on those articles for the period 1985-2004. (Since an insufficient number of up-to-date CVs were submitted by comparison group members in cycles 6 and 7, the citation analysis was carried out for just cycles 1-5.)

Data on extramural funding. To measure the extent of extramural funding received by Scholars and comparison group members, the committee examined the number of NIH grants received by them. Generally speaking, for biomedical scientists, NIH is the largest and most important source of extramural funds. Obtaining an R01 grant is considered an important rite of passage for biomedical researchers. Also data on the number and type of NIH grants are listed in the Computer Retrieval of Information on Science Projects (CRISP) database (National Institutes of Health, 2006a). NRC staff searched the CRISP database for the relevant 10 years for each Scholar and comparison group member to obtain data on the number and type of NIH grants.

The committee used these three quantitative data sources to obtain 12 outcome variables to track the progress of Scholars and comparison group members. These outcome variables are:

1. Current rank—if in academia—and prestige of academic institution.
2. Tenure status
3. Number of years to tenure
4. Current position (if not in academia)
5. Years to current position
6. Number of honors and awards
7. Number of journal articles
8. Number of citations
9. Total number of NIH grants
10. Number of years to obtain first NIH grant

11. Number of R01 grants
12. Number of years to obtain first R01 grant

Qualitative Information

Extant data collected by the Markey Trust on Markey Scholars and candidates for the award. The Markey Trustees collected a great deal of information from all the Markey Scholars and a lesser quantity of data from unsuccessful candidates for the award. At a minimum, these data consisted of the application package described earlier. For Scholars, additional data elements consisted of annual progress reports, equipment and supply expense statements, correspondence with the Trust's Miami office, and comments and assessments from the Scholar Selection Committee. Further information was available from the archived records of the Lucille P. Markey Charitable Trust Records.[1]

Ethnographic interviews of all Scholars and comparison group members conducted approximately 10 years after the assumption of the first professional position. The committee recognized that it was not possible to determine the critical decision points or the thought processes that led to those decisions from CV analysis or citation data alone. Consequently, the committee decided to conduct a relatively short—35 to 45 minute—telephone interview with all Markey Scholars and comparison group members. These interviews were conducted by a consultant who was a biomedical scientist and also trained in interviewing techniques. All interviews were recorded and transcribed. Rather than use a structured interview schedule, the committee elected to conduct ethnographic interviews[2] (Spradley, 1983).

---

[1]As the Trust was entering its final years, it arranged for all Trust documents to be archived at the Rockefeller Archive Center in Sleepy Hollow, New York. Following the conclusion of the Trust in 1997, all documents were transferred to the center, classified, and microfilmed. The archived Lucille P. Markey Charitable Trust Records currently consist of 153 reels of microfilm with approximately 800 frames on each reel. They are a rich source of information on all aspects of the Trust and will be made available to the public in 2007.

[2]Ethnographic interviews employ descriptive and structural questions. Descriptive questions are broad and general and allow people to describe their experiences, their daily activities, and objects and people in their lives. These descriptions provide the interviewer with a general idea of how individuals see their world. Structural questions are used to explore responses to descriptive questions. They are used to understand how the respondent organizes knowledge. Interviews begin with descriptive questions. Responses to the descriptive questions enable the interviewer to discover what is important to the subject and lead to structural questions. Good ethnographic interviews use the following six guidelines:

1. Ask for use instead of meaning.
2. Use open-ended questions rather than dichotomous questions that trigger a yes or no response.
3. Restate what the client says by repeating the client's exact words; do not paraphrase or interpret.

TABLE 3-1 Schedule of Markey Scholar and Comparison Group
Interviews

Markey Cycle	Year																			
	1985	1986	1987	1988	1989	1990	1991	1992	1993	1994	1995	1996	1997	1998	1999	2000	2001	2002	2003	2004
Cycle 1																				
Cycle 2																				
Cycle 3																				
Cycle 4																				
Cycle 5																				
Cycle 6																				
Cycle 7																				

Scholars and comparison group members were classified into cohorts
corresponding to the award cycles of Markey Scholars. They were interviewed approximately 10 years after they achieved their first professional
position (i.e., as an assistant professor if they remained in academia)
which was assumed to have occurred within four years of the point in
time in which an individual received or would have received the Markey
Scholar Award. These intervals were based on the committee's analysis of
the postdoctoral experience of Scholars and were designed to ensure that
all Scholars had completed their postdoctoral experience and assumed
a professorial or professional position. In practice, Scholars' years in the
postdoctorate ranged from 1 to 4 years, so the interviews were completed
approximately 14 years after they received the Markey Award. For comparison group members, the intervals were similar: 3 or 4 years in the
postdoctorate followed by 10 years of work. Therefore, all Scholars and
comparison group members were interviewed at approximately the same
time in the progression of their career and had the same number of years
to achieve rank, publish, and obtain extramural funding. In Table 3-1, we
show the start and end points for the range of years (cycle=light gray) and
the year interviewed for each of the seven cycles (indicated in the darker
gray) of Markey Scholars (and comparison groups).

---

    4. Avoid double-barreled or multiple questions.
    5. Avoid leading questions that tend to orient the person to respond in a particular
direction.
    6. Avoid using "why" questions.

Analysis of the ethnographic interviews gave the committee a more nuanced view of the pathways Scholars and comparison group members chose. The interview tracked information in 12 categories:

1. The effect of Markey award on independence as a postdoctoral fellow.
2. The effect of the Markey award on the Scholar's future plans when they were postdoctoral fellows.
3. What factors influenced the first academic position.
4. Experiences as a junior faculty member compared with those who did not have immediate support.
5. The influence the Markey award played on future funding opportunities.
6. Expectations for teaching responsibilities at first faculty position.
7. Size and composition of lab.
8. The effect of the Markey award on networking capabilities.
9. Impact on patents, licenses, commercial interests or consultancies.
10. Current and future interests in biomedical research.
11. Retrospective analysis of current research and status.
12. Orientation towards clinical research.

The focus of the interview questions was tailored specifically for Markey Scholars and comparison group members. Copies of the interview schedules used for both groups are found in Appendix F.

RESPONSE FROM SCHOLARS AND COMPARISON GROUP MEMBERS

The response to our efforts to collect CVs from and interview Scholars was almost 100 percent. With a small number of exceptions, we were able to obtain the information we sought from nearly all of the Scholars. This was expected as these individuals have had a strong connection to the Markey program over the years and our attempts to follow up with them occurred at approximately five years after the end of their Markey support.

The effort to collect information from comparison group members, by contrast, was more difficult. There were 177 nominees who were reviewed and top-ranked (the first comparison group) and 209 nominees who were classified as competitive but not top-ranked (the second comparison group). NRC staff attempted to contact all of these nominees who were reviewed by the Scholar Selection Committee. The services of Equifax, a credit reporting agency, were used to obtain current contact information for reviewed nominees. Equifax was able to supply some

TABLE 3-2 Number of Comparison Group Members, by Level of Contact

Level of Contact	Top-Ranked Candidates	Competitive Candidates	Total
Total number of reviewed nominees	177	209	386
Number with some contact data	140	154	294
Number who responded to staff inquiry	99	96	195
Number who submitted recent data	63	64	127
Number who were interviewed	51	50	101

current information—home address and/or home telephone number—on 294 (76 percent) of reviewed nominees—140 from top-ranked candidates and 154 from competitive candidates (Table 3-2). The Equifax inquiry was compromised because social security numbers were not available for any comparison group members from the first cycle of nominations and Equifax depends on the social security number to identify unique persons. As a consequence, the number of locatable persons from the first cycle of nominations for both top-ranked candidates and competitive candidates was much lower than anticipated and lower than for any other cycle. NRC staff attempted to obtain current location information on the candidates who could not be located by Equifax by using web searches and checking for affiliations of authors in relevant journals. This effort proved to be futile as only a few nominees could be accurately located and only three of the nominees who could be located responded to our inquiry; all three of those were from the top-ranked candidate group.

NRC staff attempted to contact these 294 comparison group members with moderate success. Successful contact—verifying current status and location, describing the evaluation of the Scholars and its importance for future funding policy in the biomedical sciences, and requesting participation in the evaluation—was made with 195 comparison group members (66 percent). For approximately half of the 99 nonrespondents (n = 48), the contact information we received from Equifax was incorrect (e.g., postmaster returns). Consequently, we had contact information for 99 top-ranked candidates and 96 competitive candidates. These 195 persons formed the basis for our comparison groups.

All 195 comparison group members returned current status data and, at least initially, agreed to participate in the evaluation: to submit a CV and participate in an ethnographic interview. But in fact, only 127 (66 percent) of the comparison group members actually submitted a CV and only 101 were interviewed. We were able to get some data—a CV and/or interview—from 127 of the 195 comparison group members for whom we had contact information. The percentage of top-ranked and competitive candidates interviewed out of the total number of candidates (the cooperation rate) is 29 and 24 percent respectively.

The committee recognizes that the lower than desired response rate for top-ranked and competitive candidates might affect the validity of the evaluation. Also, the committee is especially concerned about the very low number of candidates in the initial cycles of Markey funding. These very low numbers preclude potential analyses by funding cycle.

The committee recognizes the possibility of a selection bias in the two comparison groups in that some top-ranked and competitive candidates were not available to participate in the study. Unfortunately, the committee did not have the resources to contact a sample of these nonrespondents to determine if their characteristics were similar to the characteristics of those comparison group members who did respond. However, the committee reasoned that professionally successful comparison group members would be less likely to self-select out of the study.

The committee also worried that the lower than expected number of female Scholars and comparison group members may have had some impact on the study. The percentage of females at all stages of the Markey Pathway (Table 2-4) was lower than expected. In 1988 (the middle of the Markey award period), for example, 37 percent of persons graduating with doctorates in the biological sciences were female, while only 24 percent of candidates for the Markey award were female (National Science Foundation, 1997). The committee was less concerned about the higher number of candidates with Ph.D. degrees than those with M.D. or M.D./Ph.D. degrees. In 1988, there were over 4,000 Ph.D. graduates in biological sciences (National Science Foundation, 1997). However, of the nearly 16,000 M.D.s that graduated in 1988, only 214 were in M.D./Ph.D. programs and only 540 anticipated a research fellowship (American Association of Medical Colleges, 1988).

The committee is aware that the outcome measures used in this study may have been affected by both the low response rates of persons in the two comparison groups and the lower than expected number of females among Markey Scholar candidates. The latter factor, however, would not have influenced the analytical comparisons since the percent of Markey Scholars who are women (19.5%) is similar to the percent of women in each of the two comparison groups (18.8%), as shown in Table 2-4.

4

Outcomes for the Markey Scholars

ANALYSES OF CVs, CRISP, AND CITATION DATA

For the analysis of CVs, CRISP information, and citations, data were available for a total of 240 individuals in the study: 113 Scholars, 63 top-ranked candidates, and 64 competitive candidates. Of these, 80 percent were employed in academic institutions 10 years after completing their postdoctorate. For the results of the analyses of CVs, CRISP, and citation data presented in this report, the .05 level of significance is used.

Career Progression

Interestingly, Markey Scholars had held significantly more postdoctoral fellowships than top-ranked or competitive candidates. The Scholars had an average of 1.4 postdoctoral fellowships, compared to 1.1 and 1.2 for top-ranked and competitive candidates. Across all three groups, however, there was no significant difference in the time spent as a postdoctoral fellow (mean = 4.6 years). A number of Scholars considered the requirement by the Markey Trustees for at least one additional postdoctoral year to be an unreasonable burden and suggested that this requirement be dropped for any future funding vehicle for biomedical researchers.

Just under a quarter (n = 26) of the Markey Scholars were not employed in academic institutions at the time of their interview. Most of the Markey Scholars not in academia were employed in the biotech industry (n = 11), research institutes (n = 11), or at NIH (n = 2). One Scholar was practicing law and another was not in the labor force.

TABLE 4-1 Differences Among Markey Scholars, Top-Ranked, and Competitive Candidates in Academia on Selected Outcome Measures

Outcome Measure	Markey Scholar	Top-Ranked Candidate	Competitive Candidate	Significant Difference
Number	87	55	49	—
Percentage Promoted and Tenured	100	63	57	Yes[a]
Percentage in Top-Tier Universities	60	24	10	Yes[a]

[a]Markey Scholars are significantly different from both top-ranked and competitive candidates.

TABLE 4-2 Number and Percentage of Markey Scholars and Top-Ranked and Competitive Candidates in Academia by Faculty Rank

Academic Rank	Markey Scholars	Top-Ranked Candidates	Competitive Candidates	Total
Assistant Professor	0 (0%)	17 (31%)	11 (22%)	28 (15%)
Associate Professor	43 (49%)	29 (53%)	22 (45%)	94 (49%)
Professor	44 (51%)	6 (11%)	6 (12%)	56 (29%)
Other Position[a]	0 (0%)	3 (5%)	10 (20%)	13 (7%)
Total	87 (100%)	55 (100%)	49 (100%)	191 (100%)

[a]Other positions include adjunct professor, instructor, research professor, visiting professor, clinical professor, etc.

As shown in Table 4-1, of the Markey Scholars employed in academia, all were employed in tenure-track positions and all were tenured. Moreover, as shown in Table 4-2, half had also been promoted to full professor. For top-ranked and competitive candidates, not all of the academicians were in tenure-track positions, about one-quarter had not been tenured, and only a few had been promoted to full professor.

Markey Scholars in academia were also granted tenure in significantly less time than either top-ranked or competitive candidates. Markey Scholars reached tenure significantly faster with an average of 5.4 years in the professoriate, compared to 7.1 and 7.8 years for top-ranked and competitive candidates.

As also shown in Table 4-1, of the 87 Markey Scholars employed in academia, significantly more, 60 percent, were employed in "top-tier" institutions, compared to top-ranked candidates employed in academia, only 34 percent, and competitive candidates, 26 percent. We operationally defined top-tier institutions as the top-ten highest ranked institutions in the fields of biochemistry and molecular biology, cell and developmental biology, molecular and general genetics, and neurosciences as listed in Research-Doctorate Program in the United States.[1]

Publications and Citations

To examine the productivity of Scholars relative to the comparison groups, the committee calculated the number of journal articles each individual published for a 14-year period beginning with year the individual became or would have become a Markey Scholar. The 14-year period was chosen because it was assumed that all individuals would have obtained their first professional position (i.e., an assistant professorship if in academia) within four years and the focus of the assessment was on productivity from the time of the award through the period 10 years after the first professional position. Thus, for example, journal articles for those in the first cycle were counted for the period 1985-1998. Reviews in journals were not counted and neither were book chapters. The source of the data for the number of journal articles were CVs obtained from each individual included in the study (cycles 6 and 7 were excluded from this analysis due to an insufficient number of up-to-date CVs for individuals in the comparison groups). Mean and median number of articles were calculated for each group within a cycle and overall.

As shown in Table 4-3, Scholars were slightly more productive than the individuals in the two comparison groups. While top-ranked and competitive candidates had roughly the same number of mean journal articles at 36.5 and 34.8 respectively over the 14-year period, Scholars had a higher mean number of journal articles during the period at 44.1, or better than 3.1 articles per year.

There tended to be several Scholars in each cycle who were highly productive. To adjust for this, the committee also calculated the median number of journal articles per individual. As also shown in Table 4-3, top-ranked candidates had the lowest median number of journal articles,

---

[1]These institutions include, in alphabetical order: California Technological Institute; Columbia University; Harvard University; Johns Hopkins University; Massachusetts Institute of Technology; Rockefeller University; Stanford University; University of California, Berkeley; University of California, San Diego; University of California, San Francisco; University of Washington; University of Wisconsin; Washington University; and Yale University.

TABLE 4-3 Mean and Median Number of Journal Articles for Markey Scholars, Top-Ranked Candidates, and Competitive Candidates, by Cycle and Overall

Cycle	Years of Articles	Number with Article Data		
		Markey Scholars	Top-Ranked Candidates	Competitive Candidates
1	1985-1998	16	2	10
2	1986-1999	14	7	12
3	1987-2000	16	5	5
4	1988-2001	16	9	6
5	1989-2002	15	9	4
ALL		77	32	37

Cycle	Years of Articles	Mean Number of Articles		
		Scholars	Top-Ranked	Competitive
1	1985-1998	60.4	23.0	39.4
2	1986-1999	30.7	28.9	31.6
3	1987-2000	40.8	40.0	28.4
4	1988-2001	45.9	27.6	46.0
5	1989-2002	40.9	52.4	24.5
ALL		44.1	36.5	34.8

Cycle	Years of Articles	Median Number of Articles		
		Scholars	Top-Ranked	Competitive
1	1985-1998	44.5	23.0	40.0
2	1986-1999	31.5	27.0	33.0
3	1987-2000	43.0	29.0	25.0
4	1988-2001	37.0	24.0	51.5
5	1989-2002	39.0	54.0	24.5
ALL		36.0	30.0	34.0

with competitive candidates higher and Scholars just slightly higher than them.

In sum, the committee concludes that, overall, Scholars were slightly more productive than individuals in the comparison groups as measured by number of journal articles. However, much of the greater productivity was generated by Scholars in particular cycles, (e.g., 1 and 4) where several Scholars were so productive as to elevate the mean number of articles above the typical number (the median) for Scholars in that cycle.

To assess the impact of these journal articles, the committee also counted the number of citations for them through 2004. So, for cycle 1 individuals, for example, the committee tallied the citations for the period

1985-2004 for the journal articles published by this group in the period 1985-1998. For cycle 5, to provide another example, the committee counted the citations for 1989-2004 for journal articles published by individuals in this cycle during the period 1989-2002. The source of the data for the number of journal articles were CVs obtained from each individual included in the study (cycles 6 and 7 were excluded from this analysis due to an insufficient number of up-to-date CVs for individuals in the comparison groups) and citation data for each of the articles obtained from a custom database provided by the Institute for Scientific Information (ISI). Mean and median citations per individual and mean citations per article were calculated for each group within each cycle.

In addition to having higher numbers of journal articles, as shown in Table 4-4, Scholars had both higher numbers of mean and median citations per individual and higher numbers of citations per article than the individuals in the two comparison groups for almost every cycle and overall. Top-ranked candidates had higher mean and median citations than the candidates in the competitive group in three out of the five cycles and overall and higher citations per article in four of the five cycles.

Table 4-4 also shows that, as the median number of citations per individual tended to be lower than the mean number for almost every group, there were individuals, particularly among the Scholars, who elevated the mean because their articles were so highly cited. That is, the impact of some Scholars was significantly greater even than other Scholars.

Extramural Funding

One of the most important indicators of independence in the sciences is the ability to attract extramural funding. For biomedical scientists, the National Institutes of Health (NIH) is the largest and most significant provider of extramural funding. In 1996, for example, NIH awarded more than 30,000 grants totaling in excess of $8 billion. Of the awards available from the NIH, the traditional research project (R01) grant is widely accepted as the most important indicator of scientific independence. During the five-year interval from 1992 to 1996, NIH averaged 18,000 R01 awards totaling about $4 billion annually (NIH, 2006a). Using the NIH's CRISP database (National Institutes of Health, 2006b), we examined the grant productivity for all Scholars and candidate groups, regardless of their current position. We undertook this analysis both including and excluding individuals not currently employed in academia as NIH research grants are not limited to university-based researchers. We examined grant productivity from four perspectives. First, we tallied the total number of grants obtained during the 10-year interval of interest. Second, we calculated the interval between obtaining faculty status and the first NIH grant. Third, we tallied the

TABLE 4-4 Mean and Median Number of Citations per Individual and Mean Citations per Article for Markey Scholars, Top-Ranked Candidates, and Competitive Candidates

Cycle	Years of Articles	Years of Citations	Number with Citation Data		
			Scholars	Top-Ranked	Competitive
1	1985-1998	1985-2004	16	2	10
2	1986-1999	1986-2004	12	7	10
3	1987-2000	1987-2004	16	5	5
4	1988-2001	1988-2004	15	7	6
5	1989-2002	1989-2004	15	8	3
ALL			74	29	34

Cycle	Years of Articles	Years of Citations	Mean Citations per Individual		
			Scholars	Top-Ranked	Competitive
1	1985-1998	1985-2004	4,141	401	1,095
2	1986-1999	1986-2004	2,593	1,961	1,822
3	1987-2000	1987-2004	5,133	2,448	1,114
4	1988-2001	1988-2004	3,596	1,210	2,311
5	1989-2002	1989-2004	3,223	2,869	828
ALL			3,808	2,007	1,503

Cycle	Years of Articles	Years of Citations	Median Citations		
			Scholars	Top-Ranked	Competitive
1	1985-1998	1985-2004	3,200	401	1,004
2	1986-1999	1986-2004	2,261	549	1,643
3	1987-2000	1987-2004	4,003	2,176	584
4	1988-2001	1988-2004	1,733	1,299	922
5	1989-2002	1989-2004	2,381	2,486	586
ALL			2,475	1,426	980

Cycle	Years of Articles	Years of Citations	Mean Citations Per Article		
			Scholars	Top-Ranked	Competitive
1	1985-1998	1985-2004	69	17	28
2	1986-1999	1986-2004	85	68	59
3	1987-2000	1987-2004	126	61	39
4	1988-2001	1988-2004	79	51	50
5	1989-2002	1989-2004	79	53	38
ALL			86	55	43

number of R01 grants. Fourth we calculated the interval between obtaining faculty status and getting the R01. The results are shown in Tables 4-5 and 4-6. The results were generally the same whether the analysis was of all individuals or limited to those in academia.

During the ten years following their first professional position, Scholars obtained significantly more NIH grants than competitive candidates but about the same number as top-ranked candidates. There was little difference in the time to first NIH grant among the three groups. Similarly, Scholars received significantly more R01 grants than competitive candidates, though only slightly more than top-ranked candidates. Importantly, they took significantly less time to get their first R01 grant than either top-ranked or competitive candidates.

TABLE 4-5 Differences in Grant Awards Among Markey Scholars, Top-Ranked Candidates, and Competitive Candidates

Outcome Measure	Markey Scholar	Top-Ranked Candidate	Competitive Candidate	Significant Difference
Number of NIH Grants	3.3	3.2	1.9	Yes[a]
Years to First NIH Grant	3.5	4.1	3.9	No
Number of R01 Grants	1.8	1.5	0.9	Yes[a]
Years to First R01 Grant	4.0	5.6	5.6	Yes[b]

[a]Markey Scholars are significantly different from competitive candidates only.
[b]Markey Scholars are significantly different from both top-ranked and competitive candidates.

TABLE 4-6 Differences in Grant Awards Among Markey Scholars, Top-Ranked Candidates, and Competitive Candidates in Academia

Outcome Measure	Markey Scholar	Top-Ranked Candidate	Competitive Candidate	Significant Difference
Number of NIH Grants	3.5	3.4	2.2	Yes[a]
Years to First NIH Grant	3.4	3.9	3.8	No
Number of R01 Grants	2.0	1.6	1.1	Yes[b]
Years to First R01 Grant	4.0	5.4	5.5	Yes[a]

[a]Markey Scholars are significantly different from competitive candidates only.
[b]Markey Scholars are significantly different from both top-ranked and competitive candidates.

Summary

In conclusion, Scholars were significantly more likely to be promoted, tenured and work at a top-tier university. They had a higher mean number of journal articles and a slightly higher median number of journal articles. The Scholars' citations, on average, were higher both per article and per individual. While Scholars obtained significantly more NIH grants, and R01s in particular, than competitive candidates, there was no statistical difference when comparing Scholars and top-ranked candidates. However, Scholars were able to obtain R01 grants faster than both top-ranked and competitive candidates. The committee believes that the high level of productivity, especially of the top-ranked candidates, is a testament to the effectiveness of the selection process in identifying highly competitive candidates.

INTERVIEWS OF SCHOLARS AND TOP-RANKED AND COMPETITIVE CANDIDATES

We conducted 35 to 45 minute phone interviews with each of the Scholars and comparison group members approximately 10 to 12 years after they received or applied for the Markey Award. The topics in the survey instrument specifically probed the Scholar's decision-making process over those years. The ethnographic interview schedule was modified for use with the top-ranked and competitive candidates and is included in Appendix F. The committee elected to treat the interview data as descriptive; therefore, these data were not analyzed statistically.

Specifically, the interview was designed to address the following areas:

• Was the flexibility of Markey funding important? Did it enable Scholars to change locations when appropriate?
• The ability of Scholars to venture into a "risky" research agenda.
• The impact of Trustee negotiations with employing institutions to ensure that Scholars were not burdened with teaching and administrative responsibilities.
• The length of the Scholars award and the value of mandating some postdoctoral experience.
• The importance of (up to) seven years of stable funding on the family formation of biomedical scholars and their (frequently also professional) spouses.

Nomination for Markey Award

All candidates had to go through an internal institutional review process before being nominated as only six nominations per institution were permitted each year (except during the initial year, when the limit was four nominations per institutions). Sixty-four percent of the Scholars (76.2 percent of females and 61.4 percent of males) remembered being selected by their advisor or department chair to apply for the Markey Award. The remainder remembered being self-motivated in submitting their application or did not remember the process at all.

Some Scholars reported occasional "tension" between them and other postdoctoral fellows or others in the laboratory who did not get such a prestigious award, but in general the Scholars were coming from well-supported laboratories, so jealousy was rarely an issue.

Independence

Approximately 60 percent of the Scholars considered themselves independent at the time they received the Markey award in terms of their capacity to devise their own experiments prior to starting their post-doctoral or fellow position. The remaining Scholars felt that their sense of independence developed during this period.

Differences in the self-report of independence, however, were dependent on the group, the academic degree, and the gender of the respondents. Among Ph.D.s, Scholars claimed independence at a higher rate than top-ranked and competitive candidates. Scholars who were Ph.D.s reported feeling more independent than M.D.s or M.D./Ph.D.s. in the other two groups (Table 4-7). Female Scholars were less likely to report being independent at the start of their postdoctorate than were the males and Ph.D. (Table 4-8). Females in the top-ranked candidate pool, however, reported a greater sense of independence than the female Markey Scholars, but the sample sizes were too small to provide conclusive results. More males among competitive candidates reported a developing period of independence than Markey Scholar males.

TABLE 4-7 Percentage Claiming Independence, by Degree and Group

	Ph.D.	M.D., & M.D./Ph.D.	Total
Scholars	67 (n = 42)	40 (n = 27)	61 (n = 69)
Top-ranked	46 (n = 17)	71 (n = 10)	53 (n = 17)
Competitive	42 (n = 13)	32 (n = 6)	38 (n = 19)
Total	55 (n = 72)	50 (n = 43)	53 (n = 115)

TABLE 4-8 Percentage Claiming Independence, by Gender and Group

	Male	Female	Total
Scholars	65 (n = 59)	42 (n = 10)	61 (n = 69)
Top-ranked	50 (n = 21)	47 (n = 6)	53 (n = 27)
Competitive	34 (n = 13)	50 (n = 6)	38 (n = 19)
Total	54 (n = 93)	50 (n = 22)	53 (n = 115)

Several Scholars mentioned that they appreciated having the extra time in their postdoctoral period (as stipulated by the Markey Award) to develop new lines of investigation and to cement their independence from their postdoctoral mentor. For many Scholars, having their own supply money and salary meant that those Scholars were able to function as a sort of "lab within a lab" in the latter days of their postdoctoral appointments.

The top-ranked and competitive candidates used a variety of alternate support mechanisms to fund their postdoctoral training period. The majority of top-ranked candidates (66 percent) had support from either HHMI or private non-profit foundations. The majority of competitive candidates (48 percent), in contrast, had support through government training grants (either NRSAs or medical school residency/fellowship support). Other forms of support for both groups included using the PI's research grant funds or international government support. In all cases, the support was usually for salary only or with at best very small allotments for supplies. Ninety percent of the top-ranked candidates and 84 percent of the competitive candidates, however, reported they did not have to cut short their postdoctoral training due to a lack of funding.

Very few Scholars commented that they changed their research direction after receiving the award, but many mentioned the award (and the time that came with it) gave them the confidence to pursue "riskier" lines of research.

> I think the Markey money encouraged the fellows to take more risks and thus impacted on research productivity - many of us had a poor production rate with papers during our postdoctoral fellowships because we were trying new things. However, most of the Markeys were very creative and spontaneous in their work, which I see as the most important thing. (Scholar)

> The Markey gave me a lot of bullets and I could just start shooting and some of the bullets hit! All in all, the Markey Award was wonderful because it allowed me to be less methodological, less reliant on validation, and I had very little

hindrance in terms of scientific questions. I had less pressure to produce, but ended up producing a lot as a result! (Scholar)

The strength of the program was that they supported true innovation, not just variations on a theme; I have never found that since. (Scholar)

I do believe, given the nature and abilities of the Markey scholars who were selected, they would have done fine regardless. These were the blue chip investments. Still, maybe in this day and age, we should also think about the mavericks out there, the ones willing to do things at even a higher risk level. (Scholar)

Knowing that I had five years of support made it easy for me to decide to pursue research that would otherwise have been very difficult to fund. I think that aspect of the Markey is something that is so valuable. My science career would have been very different without it, and would have made much less impact. (Scholar)

Comments from the comparison group members emphasize the ability of Scholars to be innovative, by highlighting how conservative one might be otherwise.

There are a "whole group of guys, like myself, who were raised in a time when you had to be really conservative and grant proposals had to be backed with a lot of data. It carries over into our approaches now; we are really still very conservative in our proposals to get NIH money because of the hard times in our past. We got shell-shocked. (Top-Ranked Candidate)

NIH should set aside 10-15 percent of their funds for high-risk experiments (as NCI does). NIH should fund research where if it works, it would really pay off. Look at Maya Lin (architect for the Vietnam Memorial), if she had been submitting a grant to NIH she wouldn't have a chance because of her lack of experience. NIH should be funding the idea, not the work record. (Competitive Candidate)

Awareness came for me when I tried to write the Markey application. I was supposed to write something innovative, and I realized I couldn't do it. I realized I was a product of a myopic way of doing science and I couldn't break out of it. (Competitive Candidate)

The attitude of many who were among the top-ranked or competitive candidates was highlighted by one who stated:

The separation between being a success and being a disaster is razor thin. I am fortunate that I have a good position, a lab, am funded. I can see how a different fork in the path could have led to very different circumstances. I would like to think that some of the branch points didn't go my way, but through effort, determination, skill and talent I managed to take another fork to get things done. I can't give up; I have to keep going. Abe Lincoln said "people are about as happy as they make up their minds to be." Rejection is not pleasant; not getting the Markey did take its toll. I had worked with big name people, was used to getting papers accepted on the first pass, and getting rewarded all along the way. Suddenly this wasn't happening and it took the wind out of my sails. (Candidate)

Transition from Postdoctoral or Fellow Status to First Professional Position

When asked about their job search process, many Scholars commented that they were invited to apply for positions by members of the Markey Selection committee or by individuals who were speakers at the Markey Scholar annual meetings. Many of the Scholars noted that they had several job offers, sometimes more than five at a time. Variables influencing the Scholar's assessment of the attractiveness of a particular job offer included spouse's job requirements, quality of graduate student population, research interests, reputation of the department, as well as the cost of living in a specific geographical region (Table 4-9).

By contrast, candidates mentioned the quality of science as a deciding factor only 46 percent of the time, less than for Scholars, 70 percent of whom cited the quality of science as a determining factor. It seems likely that the job hunt was more stressful for the candidates than for the Scholars.

The award gave me an enormous sense of security. It encouraged me to focus my job search on the thing that I would really like, and to take a very long-term view. (Scholar)

Forty applications, two interviews, two job offers. (Candidate)

TABLE 4-9 Percentage Distribution of Reasons for Selecting First Professional Position, by Group

Reason[a]	Scholars	Top-ranked Candidates	Competitive Candidates
Quality of Science	70	57	35
Family Issues	33	30	25
Geography	24	24	9
Quality of Graduate Students	12	3	3

[a]Respondents could list multiple reasons.

Approximately 40 percent of respondents from the competitive candidate group commented that economic factors played a large role in their decision in that they only had one job offer and they had to take it.

A number of Scholars also volunteered that the award gave dual scientific career couples time to get "in sync" with differing career stages and also allowed for more flexibility when it came to looking for positions for dual career couples. Thirty percent of the Scholars stated the flexibility of the award (length of postdoctoral training, choice of institutions) meant that they felt they had much less of a problem finding a position amenable to both parties.

> *I would say that was the single greatest effect that the Markey had on our lives: the Award gave us that fluidity where I could maintain postdoctoral status until my wife was ready to enter the job market. (Scholar)*

> *One of the most important things was that it allowed my husband and me to start a family; I think everybody in my year had babies; the director said "they are spawning like fish out there." Give a 30-year old a six-year grant, and the first thing they are going to do is have a baby. It was much easier for a married couple looking for two faculty positions to find two tenure-track positions. We both were able to take good jobs. (Scholar)*

> *Markey babies . . . you had some security; your life won't be uprooted right away. I was worried they would think I wasn't serious about her career. Later I noticed that almost every woman that year had children, one had twins. (Scholar)*

> *I ended up spending about 2.5 years as a fellow, followed by a "semi-down time" year to start a family. I chose (university) because my parents were there and I wanted to be close to family and my spouse liked the area and didn't want to move. (Scholar)*

In contrast, approximately 30 percent of the candidates noted they had a significant two-body problem when it came to finding positions after the completion of their training.

> *We needed a job for both: one would follow the other. (Candidate)* ·

Individuals with a Ph.D. were far more likely to change institutions after the completion of their postdoctoral training period than those who had either an M.D. or M.D./Ph.D. degree. When M.D.s or M.D./Ph.D.s were queried as to why they opted to stay at their fellowship institutions despite the typical lack of startup funds, several clinical Scholars cited that the deciding factor was that they were "intertwined" in a support system

TABLE 4-10 Number Who Changed Institutions Between the Completion of Training and Commencement of First Faculty Appointment, by Group and Degree

	Scholars	Top-ranked Candidates	Competitive Candidates
M.D.	7	1	2
M.D./Ph.D.	15	5	5
Ph.D.	49	28	19

at the fellowship institution that would be difficult to replicate at a new institution (Table 4-10).

> *I was able to "hit the ground running" by staying on at (top-tier university), rather than pursuing a career elsewhere. (Scholar)*

> *My reasons for staying were partly personal, and partly because I had such a strong network of people to interact with that it seemed like it would be a very good, supportive environment. (Scholar)*

> *The award smoothed the transition while I was juggling clinical loads. (Scholar)*

Scholars reported that startup packages for those who stayed at their fellowship or postdoctoral institution were less than packages for those who moved to new institutions. Some Scholars reported uncomfortable negotiations with their future department chairs who tried to reduce packages because Markey Award funds were seen as filling the need, and that they would have really appreciated some additional guidance from the Markey Committee members.

It was at this transition point, from fellowship to first professional position, that many individuals considered leaving academic bench science. Many of these individuals reported moving into the pharmaceutical or biotechnology industry, but in the Scholars group, 3 out of the 9 Ph.D.s and 1 of the 4 M.D.s who left academic science went to work at research institutes with no academic commitments, and 1 of the 7 M.D./Ph.D.s took a position at NIH (Table 4-11). The remaining Scholars left academic bench science to establish companies in the biotechnology industry or to work in pharmaceutical companies. Many of these Scholars who left academia are senior executives in the biotechnology industry today. Some individuals from all three groups left the traditional science arena completely and went into very diverse occupations such as patent law, home-making, pottery-making, or legislative affairs.

TABLE 4-11 Number who Left Academic Bench Science by the Time of Interview, by Group

	Scholars	Top-ranked Candidates	Competitive Candidates
Total	20	6	16
M.D.	4	2	2
M.D./Ph.D.	7	1	2
Ph.D.	9	3	12

At that time I was debating whether to remain in academia or go into industry. I applied for the Markey award. It was going to be the decision-maker. If I got the grant, I would remain in academia. (Scholar)

Faculty Years: Administrative Duties

Generally, any committee responsibilities the Scholars had were equivalent to those of other junior faculty members without their own sources of support. Many Scholars mentioned they wanted to be active members of their departments, so they volunteered for committee work. The key then was to know "when to say yes" and not overburden oneself. Some clinical Markey Scholars needed the Markey Selection Committee members to "remind" department chairs of their commitment to give Scholars 75 percent protected time for research. The candidates in both groups reported committee work loads similar to those of the Markey Scholars.

While moving into my apartment, I got two phone calls asking me to be on graduate admissions committees and to organize a symposium because they were looking for someone "just like her" (i.e., female). (Scholar)

Initially, I was overloaded with committee work, and then the Markey organization stepped in and "saved" me. (Scholar)

I think that females get asked much less often to sit on scientific advisory boards, and in general perhaps, are not so interested in getting into the company/ administrative side of things. (Top-Ranked Candidate)

Faculty Years: Funding

The majority of the Scholars considered the Markey award as having a positive influence on their subsequent funding efforts. But, as one Scholar said, "I never saw it mentioned on a pink sheet," meaning this isn't the sort of information provided in a NIH review (a.k.a., pink sheet) so he really had no insight into how the award affected his NIH funding award. Several Scholars felt that the award gave them a "stamp of approval," especially after the award became better known. Scholars frequently commented at this point in the interview that having the Markey Award meant they could get sufficient pilot data to submit a strong R01 proposal. That is, the award gave them time to do experiments and establish their independence prior to submitting their first NIH grant proposal.

Many of the individuals from the candidate groups commented on the difficulties of securing funding for their research programs in the early 1990's. That was a period of significant tightening in NIH funding, and, therefore, establishing a new research program was particularly challenging. Many candidates reported writing multiple grant proposals during this period and feeling extremely lucky to get one of them funded.

NIH eats their young. The R29 was critical to my career success—it gave me the self confidence when I was teetering in the balance. (Candidate)

Receiving the Physician/Scientist training award did not change my career plans but rather validated my hopes that I would have a research career. It was like a big plank that was handed to me to step up to the next thing I wanted to do. (Candidate)

Faculty Years: Teaching

Two-thirds of the Scholars reported less than a 10 percent time commitment to didactic teaching in the initial years of their faculty appointment. As the Scholars climbed the academic career ladder, they experienced more administrative responsibilities, especially an increase in teaching loads. Even 10 years after getting the award, however, the teaching responsibilities were not a significant portion of the Scholars' workload. The Scholars' teaching loads did not appear to differ from those of candidates who remained in academia. Teaching loads for top-ranked and competitive candidates were similar to those of Scholars. Scholars estimated that their mentoring or attending duties averaged around 25-30 percent of their work effort.

Scholars in academia were somewhat more likely than either candidate group to have large labs. Half of the Scholars in academia maintained moderate-sized laboratory groups of 6-10 people. Competitive candidates were evenly split between labs with less than 5 people, or labs with 6-10 people. Only four competitive candidate PIs had labs greater with more than 11 people (Table 4-12).

TABLE 4-12 Number of Principal Investigators in Academia, by
Laboratory Size and Group

Group	Laboratory Size			
	5 and Under	6 to 10	11 and Over	Total
Scholars	10	38	28	76
Top-ranked Candidates	11	9	13	33
Competitive Candidates	10	10	4	24

Many M.D.s or M.D./Ph.D.s with clinical loads had a lab manager or
senior research associate managing the labs while they were on attending
duties. Several M.D.s commented that it was difficult to get good graduate students if they were in medical departments. The Scholars' trainees
(graduate students, fellows and postdoctoral fellows) have gone into a
variety of careers: academic, biotech, industry and "other."

Networking

The Scholars repeatedly mentioned that attending the annual Scholars
meeting was a wonderful experience. The energy and enthusiasm was
infectious.

*I think in many ways the biggest strength of the program was my exposure to
other Markey Scholars at the meetings. (Scholar)*

One Scholar from an early class (Classes 1-3) noted what she called
the "cocktail party effect." That is, access to speakers and committee
members at meals and social events was a critical component to their
subsequent success. At the annual Markey meetings, Scholars got to know
people on review committees for other foundations and NIH review
panels (speakers, invited guests etc.). Several Scholars also noted that
having a name associated with a face or project was an important asset for
getting subsequent proposals to stand out and, of course, for job hunting,
as mentioned previously.

*A minor issue, which affected me and perhaps a few others in the program, was
being forced to give up the Markey meetings when I became a Hughes Investigator . . . it somehow felt very sad being kicked out. It was sad to be excluded
from the meetings. These meetings were really incredible and valuable part of
the program. (Scholar)*

Although scientific collaborations between the Markey Scholars were few (primarily it seems due to the diverse nature of the science covered), several Scholars noted they felt comfortable calling or e-mailing another Scholar for information on a technique or to invite them to a speaker series.

Commercial Interests

In the process of interviewing the early classes (Classes 1 to 3) we noticed that several Scholars mentioned starting their own businesses or other commercial interests. Many of the Scholars reported serving on Scientific Advisory Boards for biotechnology companies while maintaining their academic appointments. Starting with Class 3, we added a question to the survey instrument to assess how prevalent this observation was in reality.

Forty-three of the respondents in the Scholars group, 87 percent of them males, reported having patents or licenses. The holding of licenses or patents appears to be independent of degree.

Sixteen out of the 85 Scholars who answered the question on business interests had started their own businesses, and all of these individuals were male. The number of females in the candidate groups was small, but none of those women reported starting their own businesses.

Why don't more women sit on scientific advisory boards for biotech companies? Maybe because no one approaches them, the old boys network, or do the women decline because they are too busy with work and family? (Scholar)

M.D.s and M.D./Ph.D.s who were Scholars reported more consulting for profit than did the Ph.D.s. Many of these clinical Scholars had paid consultancies with pharmaceutical companies in the arena of drug discovery (Table 4-13). The rates of consulting did not differ between males and

TABLE 4-13 Percentage of Interviewees Engaged in Commercial Interests, by Type of Interest and Group

Group	Percentage in Commercial Interest		
	Licenses or Patents	Started a Business	Consult for Profit
Scholar	23	14	28
Top-Ranked	32	5	32
Competitive	23	8	36
Total	25	10	31

females. One hundred percent of the competitive candidate M.D./Ph.D.s (11 people) were consulting for profit, (compared with 64 percent of the M.D./Ph.D.s in the Scholars group (n = 14).

As noted above, this is probably an "underreporting" of the incidence of commercial involvement, as individuals in the first two cohorts were not specifically asked this question. It was of special interest to note that in all the categories queried, female Scholars had fewer reports of commercial interests than male Scholars. Whether the seeming under-representation of females reflected a lack of interest or a lack of opportunity or a combination of both was beyond the scope of this investigation.

Envision Statements

The interviews concluded with questions about where the Scholars had envisioned being 10 years after assuming their first professional position. Many individuals laughed and said they had no "plan" and were just immensely grateful that they had a career and a lifestyle that they enjoyed very much. Many of those who went into the biotechnology industry confessed that they would never have considered that a career option when they were staring as postdoctoral fellows. Rather, they ended up taking advantage of unexpected opportunities, or taking a risk on a new entrepreneurial venture.

> Originally, I wanted to be 100 percent academic, so the fact that I am in the biotechnology industry is wholly unexpected. (Scholar)

Scholars who had made 5- or 10-year plans claimed they advanced far more then they had anticipated. Overall, the Scholars expressed a very high level of personal satisfaction with both their careers and their lifestyles.

> I never imagined I would be where I am today; I was going to give academia a try. (Scholar)

> I never imagined being at a major research facility. Opportunities here are very different. And I am committed to teaching, which I did not anticipate when I started here. (Scholar)

In general the top-ranked candidates were also very satisfied with their career progression, although several of them mentioned being frustrated with how much time they spent writing grant proposals. Several of them commented that they had no idea that a non-academic career could be so fulfilling, and that they wished they had known it earlier. The committee observed that, generally speaking, Markey Scholars and top-ranked and competitive candidates were pretty happy with their careers

> *Running an independent research laboratory was definitely the target. However, I always imagined myself in some university or medical school—not in the position I am right now [at a Research Institute]. I think teaching is very useful for focusing the directions of the experiments. (Top-Ranked Candidate)*

> *What I am doing now is not what I envisioned. It is more cerebral and less hands-on. My life style and general satisfaction are much higher doing what I am doing now. (Top-Ranked Candidate)*

> *I want to be in a place where basic science and translational science coexist. I see the future of research as being highly multidisciplinary. I have come to appreciate that the culture differences and culture clashes between the different disciplines have slowed us down. I would like to get back to the lab bench rather than consuming my time in administration. (Top-Ranked Candidate)*

> *The scary part was that you are stepping out of a plane without a parachute. I guess this is what I thought I would be doing, but I never realized that I would be spending the majority of my time "begging for money" (writing grants) and not be in the lab so much. I really miss being in the lab. (Competitive Candidate)*

> *I would never have imagined myself where I am now. My career has been full of surprises and turns. Nowadays, when I'm mentoring people, I always tell them to have a 5-year plan. It's a nice idea which I was never able to follow. (Competitive Candidate)*

> *I always knew I would be close to an interesting and challenging area; if the funding and timing had been better, I could have held my own in academia. (Competitive Candidate)*

> *When I was a postdoctoral fellow I only thought of academia. Once I was introduced to the pharmaceutical industry, I came here without any expectations. I thought that I would be doing research at the bench much longer. I guess it was karma, fate, and serendipity that let me supervise all these people. And I think that what I do is not that far from the academic world. (Competitive Candidate)*

> *As a postdoctoral fellow at a major academic institution, you are on a high plateau of basic research; it is the be all and end all of life. I think my perspective has broadened since then. I see the research as important and something I want to do, but now I put more weight on the clinical and teaching responsibilities. I put more emphasis on seeing that the research is applied. The main difference is*

seeing the greater importance of things outside of basic research. (Competitive Candidate)

In some ways, yes, but I never get to do experiments anymore. I sit at my desk writing and reading mostly. This is somewhat disappointing and not what I was expecting; it is a very stressful existence. I never anticipated the stress, the worry, and the horrible feeling of not getting a grant. (Competitive Candidate)

If I didn't get the Markey Award, I was amenable to working in industry where I wouldn't have to spend all my time writing. If I was going to write all the time, I would want to write cheap sleazy novels and make some significant dollars doing that! (Competitive Candidate)

Practice of Medicine and Impact of Medical Training on Research

At the time of the award, 95 percent of M.D. Scholars and 60 percent of M.D./Ph.D. Scholars had active medical licenses. The remaining persons with M.D.s had never completed a residency or had completed a residency but opted not to practice medicine. At the time of the interview, 10 to 12 years later, 50 percent of the M.D.s still had active medical licenses while only 44 percent of the M.D./Ph.D.s had kept their licenses current. There appear to be two groups of Scholars who held a M.D. degree but no license: those who never got a medical license (i.e., did not complete a residency) and those who gave up the practice of medicine after concluding they were progressing well down a path to a successful basic research career.

Getting the Markey gave me the freedom not to pursue the residency. In retrospect, it may have been good for me because it meant the department couldn't pressure me to take on clinical duties. (Scholar)

I considered doing a residency for the next two or three years at the time that I applied for the Markey Award, but when I got it I decided not to pursue a residency. (Scholar)

I had not practiced medicine since before I got the Markey. . . . . I found it too distracting to bounce back and forth between the hematology/oncology clinic and laboratory. (Scholar)

I am not licensed to practiced medicine. I found it too difficult to do both medicine and research well and made a choice. It was just too difficult to juggle with a family life. (Scholar)

I think I would have been too unsatisfied knowing that I couldn't do as good a job at either one as I could do if I was focusing. (Scholar)

As time passed, the clinical work became a distraction, so I focused totally on research and gave up my license. (Scholar)

I came to the conclusion that there were just far too many doctors in this country, and I wanted to do the basic science. They'd never miss me in the clinics; but if I'm not at the lab bench things will never get done. I like the interpersonal relationships with my peers in research much better than I do in clinical research. (Scholar)

A much higher percentage of M.D.s or M.D./Ph.D.s from the candidate groups maintained active medical licenses (88 percent) when compared to clinically-trained Scholars. Several of them intimated they had maintained their licenses as either a "security blanket" or to supplement their basic research faculty salaries. It may be that the Markey award helped the Scholars to commit definitively to research careers.

I had my personal reasons not to go into the clinical field. I felt I could not achieve the maximum results in my work if I practiced both research and clinical work. I did not want to sacrifice any more family time to my work either. I also knew that I wanted to do ventures in the biotechnology industry. All in all, staying in research science was the best choice for me. (Top-Ranked Candidate)

Sometimes the clinic can be uplifting change of pace when the research isn't going so well, and it works both ways. (Top-Ranked Candidate)

My basic science career is gone; my clinical science career is going strong. I am making lemonade. I have tailored my research to my surroundings. (Top-Ranked Candidate)

In the beginning I did one month service a year—the work was 3-4 night calls a month and that work doubled my salary. I still do night calls and that makes it possible for me to do independent research as well as clinical work. (Top-Ranked Candidate)

I know practically no one in my peer group who is active clinically and doing laboratory research. Back in the '80's, when I was still a fellow, people had the idea of combining clinical work and bench research. But I think that has pretty much gone by the wayside now. (Competitive Candidate)

None of the Scholars interviewed declared that getting a medical degree was a mistake. Rather, they viewed their clinical training as making them better scientists, in that they were more "in tune" with the impact of disease on patients, and the need for research in specific areas.

My clinical training has recently influenced my research directions, however. (Scholar)

My research really impacts on my clinical work—the question is what other tools can I use to help the patients? Translational research is the driving force in my lab—the real motivation, but I have to admit that I have never got the "ah hah" feeling with the patients and then ran back to the lab to do an experiment. (Scholar)

My ultimate goal is to apply my research to patient treatment. This is always on my mind and is driving my research interests. (Scholar)

Physicians understand that medicine is an art, not a science, and that every patient is a new chance to learn. The ability to learn and adapt is the key. (Scholar)

My clinical work helps me set my priorities for my research projects. (Scholar)

As somebody who did clinical medicine part-time, I always viewed myself as somebody having a different role to play. I always saw my role as teaching fellows, residents and students to try and bridge the clinical world with the translational basic science world, and to try to provide the students with insights into the mechanisms of disease. (Scholar)

Every once in a while a clinical patient will stimulate my research ideas, but not vice versa. (Competitive Candidate)

I think my research activity makes me a better doctor. The biggest schism I've ever seen is developing between people who do science and people who do medicine. I think this is destructive. (Competitive Candidate)

It is very important for me to be an oncologist because I see how little progress we have made, and I think it makes me do better science. (Competitive Candidate)

I bring to discussions on clinical trials a real world perspective on cancer treatments. (Competitive Candidate)

If you want to do research as an M.D. in a medical school, the idea is that you had better support yourself, because it is a luxury thing that you are doing for your own fun. (Competitive Candidate)

Participation in Translational or Clinical Research

When queried about whether they participated in translational research, which the committee defined as taking findings from the bench

TABLE 4-14 Percentage of Interviewees Engaged in Clinical or Translational Research, by Group

Group	Engaged in Clinical Research[a]	Engaged in Translational Research	Planning Future Translational Research
Scholars	22	34	55
Top-Ranked	16	31	45
Competitive	28	38	50
All	22	34	52

[a]Respondents could be in engaged in all three categories of research.

to bedside and requiring Internal Review Board approvals, only 34 percent of all Scholars responded affirmatively (Table 4-14). Many of the M.D. and M.D./Ph.D. Markey Scholars, defined "doing" clinical research as advising on design and analysis, which was not categorized as an affirmative response by the committee. Few were actually heading up clinical trials, citing the daunting amount of paperwork. Even fewer Scholars, 22 percent, were actually engaged in clinical research. It is interesting to note, however, that over half of the Scholars indicated plans for future participation in translational research. Roughly the same percentage of individuals from the candidate groups were involved with patient research and clinical trials, especially those candidates who were working in pharmaceutical firms and heading up clinical trials was their primary function.

Design of the Markey Program

At the end of the interview, the Scholars were asked how they would have improved the program if it were to be offered again. Several recurring themes emerged from the final comments made by the Scholars:

1. They greatly appreciated the Trust's philosophy of "we have faith and trust in the scholar."

2. In hindsight, they were quite grateful for the lack of bureaucracy imposed by the Markey Trust and the flexibility produced by the Trust in the Scholar as opposed to an investment in a project.

3. The supportive atmosphere, even for such well qualified scientists as the Scholars, was highly appreciated and several Scholars mentioned the "pat on the back" they received at the meetings meant more than the funds.

4. The intellectual stimulation provided by the scientific meetings, even though they were frequently outside the Scholar's area of expertise,

was invigorating and prepared them for a more broad-minded approach to science.

Unrestricted funds are incredibly important for my scientific development. I didn't fully realize it until my Markey, Searle, and Packard funds were gone. (Scholar)

The program was inspired. The selection committee and Trustees clearly cared. Secondly, many career development awards don't give people sufficient funds to be independent. The intelligent part of the Markey Scholars awards was that it started with a major infusion of funds, and then wound down over the years. The fact there were no strings attached was extremely important. Whoever designed the Scholars awards understood how NIH works and doesn't work, and how people's careers are best supported. (Scholar)

I thought the Markey was really unique; the duration of support was really great and one of the things that made the Markey so special was the people who were involved in directing its operation were really outstanding. If you can get people like that together, things work and it felt great to be a part of it. The success of the Markey is the quality of the people who were running it. (Scholar)

One of the more important aspects was not the dollars but a feeling of protection in some way and camaraderie, both between the participants and the people who were in some way involved with the Markey Foundation. What I would like to convey is not just the idea that it is great to give people lots of dollars but that it is equally important to address the welfare of the scholars; money alone is not what it is about. (Scholar)

The Markey had a really positive impact. This kind of a pat on the back, keep-on-going-you're-doing-OK, really gives you courage, confidence, extra motivation to go on; it was really a positive thing in psychological terms just as much as material. (Scholar)

I really like the idea of bridge funding, and if they are looking for new funding models, I would like to see someone consider funding a person around the 4-5 year point of a junior faculty position. That is when they are on the brink of getting really interesting results, but if the person is working on a high risk project, it will be very difficult to get funding. That is the point when people are close, but not yet at the jackpot. (Scholar)

It was difficult to get the Scholars to offer constructive criticism of the program, as many responded initially that the program was ideal as it was originally designed. However, when pressed, they made the following seven suggestions for improvements:

1. Have a more formal mentoring system. Many Scholars reported a "feeling" that someone on the Markey Selection Committee was looking out for them, but they didn't know who, and some wished they could have gone to the Committee members directly for advice.

2. The additional year for postdoctoral studies should be optional. Early classes were required to spend an additional year in the postdoctoral environment. They could change laboratories, but they could not start their own labs. Several Scholars in later classes protested this requirement, and it was eventually dropped. It should be noted that when queried about the additional one-year of postdoctoral study requirement, 51 percent of the Scholars felt this was a good idea, and another 41 percent said it had no effect on their future plans. An additional 6 percent felt the extra year was a burden and petitioned the Markey committee to remove this requirement (which was done after the third class). Those who felt the additional year was a good idea cited such factors as that the extra year gave them time to finish experiments, time to collect sufficient pilot data to be competitive for NIH awards, and time to conduct a job search.

3. Provide counsel during job negotiations, especially with startup packages. Several Scholars cited the Burroughs Wellcome (Burroughs Wellcome Fund and Howard Hughes Medical Institute, 2004) job negotiation support as an ideal way to help the job applicant to assess the competitiveness of the job offer. Scholars recommended that such a system be installed in any new program.

4. The salary component could have been shifted to the equipment/ supply budget if needed. Several Scholars noted that they felt their department was getting a "free ride" and that they were especially resentful, therefore, when the department chair tried to offer a reduced startup package. Clinical Scholars noted that as they were providing clinical service, at least some of their salaries should have come from the clinical department. Several queried whether it would have created a greater sense of commitment by the department if they had paid the salaries.

5. Reduce the number of years of support to fund more Scholars. All the Scholars were extremely sad that such a wonderful program had only 7 classes. Several, who did not understand that the Trust had to be spent out within a fixed period of time, questioned whether it would it have made more sense to trim the program back to six years from seven to get more people enrolled.

6. Do not exclude Scholars who move to government, the biotechnology industry, or HHMI from attending the annual meetings, although it is appropriate to stop additional payments. Many of the Scholars who migrated to HHMI and the biotechnology industry were extremely sad to be "kicked out of the club" of Markey Scholars when they left their aca-

demic appointments. All Scholars were invited to the last Markey Meeting in Puerto Rico in 2002.

7. Encourage collaborations by providing seed-money funds. Additional funds could have been ear-marked specifically for starting collaborations between the Markey Scholars. As their research fields or even disciplines rarely overlapped, collaborations or interdisciplinary projects were difficult to start. Perhaps the addition of a competitive fund of about $50,000 per project would have lowered the barriers to these collaborations and supported innovative research lines.

During the interview process, the interviewer noticed a subtle change in tone between respondents in the first three classes, and those in subsequent classes. The earlier class members had very fond memories of the Markey program and appeared extremely grateful for the opportunity to prove their scientific merit. Subsequent classes, while still grateful, frequently expressed the opinion that if they had not received the Markey award, they would have gotten "something else" of equal value or merit; that is, the Markey award was wonderful, but it was just one of several awards for which they could have applied and would have received.

Individuals from the two candidate groups were asked to comment on what they thought would contribute to the design of a successful program with the goal of developing a person's biomedical career. The candidates suggested a new funder should consider the following six possibilities when planning funding strategies:

1. Supporting advanced postdoctoral fellows. Several of the candidates mentioned that since postdoctoral fellowships were taking longer (between 4-5 years is not atypical now), that a new funding program should consider targeting individuals in the latter years of their postdoctorate.

2. Providing merit awards for senior scientists in the future. By developing a series of "merit awards" with significant funds attached, funders could develop an excellent mechanism to stimulate innovative thinking in experienced scientists.

3. Supporting collection of pilot data for a second NIH grant with a new line of investigation. Providing funds to a mid-level scientist to start a new line of research could promote significant risk taking or innovation in this population of scientists.

4. Underwriting interdisciplinary projects. As science in the 21st century becomes more interdisciplinary, funds need to be set aside for developing projects that bring a variety of disciplines together, and enhance collaborative activities, even over geographical boundaries. A specific suggestion was to require a co-PI system, where one PI was a M.D. and the other a Ph.D. in a complementary basic science field. Numerous M.D.s and

M.D./Ph.D.s left bench science in the early 1990s during the last downturn in the NIH funding cycle. This pool of individuals may be ideally suited for this sort of co-PI project.

5. Funding more diversely so as to find the "stars." Several candidates commented that it might be a wise idea to cast the net wider when looking for applicants—that is, to consider non-conventional applications that show a lot of thought or promise and to take the risk that this person could follow through on the ideas.

6. Providing more mentoring throughout the career timeline. This is a repeating theme among both the Scholars and candidates. Many individuals felt that more explicit mentoring during the job search and early faculty years was essential, but that this mentoring should continue through to tenure if possible.

> *I guess I would give people money to play with: relax on how well matured the ideas are . . . give them money between their postdoctoral fellowship and beginning of the career that they can make mistakes with or go down blind alleys. Take the pressure off . . . let them get going without worrying about doing their most exciting research right away. (Candidate)*

> *As a "survivor" of the crash in funding of the early 90's I am especially sensitive to the needs of young faculty. . . . I was almost forced out of science due to a lack of funding in those early years, but now I consider myself truly successful. (Candidate)*

> *The ones who are really trying to move basic findings into clinical practice are the ones who need the most support. They should target additional funds to further down the career pipeline to early mid-career plus institutional reforms to provide a more stable and better environment for dual career people. (Candidate)*

> *I would perhaps like to see the pie sliced a little thinner, spread out a little bit more amongst people. One of the elements of science is the unknown—you never know who is going to do well. (Candidate)*

Candidate Comments on Markey Award

Several of the candidates used the interview period as an opportunity to declare their frustration with the Markey Award process. The Scholar Selection Committee did not provide written critiques of the application packages for unsuccessful candidates. The rejected applicants found this lack of feedback on their Markey application particularly distressing. They would have greatly appreciated a constructive rejection letter that indicated how they had scored in areas such as: quality of the scientific proposal, skills necessary to perform the experiments outlined in the scientific proposal, letters of recommendation, and productivity. The candidates believed that since they spent a significant amount of time and effort preparing a proposal, the least they could expect in return was some sort of guidance on how to improve subsequent proposals.

There were also several complaints that there appeared to be a "coast-bias" in that the majority of the awardees came from either the West or East Coast of the United States, and that this in some way was a form of cherry-picking. The third theme that appeared was that there was an apparent lack of diversity in the awardees; nearly all Scholars were white males.

5

Lucille P. Markey
Visiting Fellows Program

In September, 1984, the Markey Trustees met with leading biomedical scientists in the United Kingdom to explore the possibility of establishing a program to support a small number of outstanding, young biomedical scientists from the United Kingdom who would spend two years pursuing their research in a leading biomedical institution in the United States. This program was proposed in recognition of the support the Medical Research Council (MRC) afforded researchers from the United States. In addition, the Trustees recognized the impact of the cutbacks in support available in the United Kingdom through the MRC. Following subsequent discussions in 1985, the Trustees finalized a plan to fund United Kingdom scholars in United States institutions. Later, the Visiting Fellows program was expanded to include Visiting Fellows from Australia. A total of 36 Visiting Fellows—26 United Kingdom Visiting Fellows and 10 Australian Visiting Fellows—were awarded support between 1986 and 1994. Total support for the Visiting Fellows program amounted to $3,298,000. The Visiting Fellows Program had a number of salient features:

- Four two-year awards would be made in each of three years beginning in July, 1986, for a total of 12 awards. In the initial year, each awardee would receive a stipend of $25,000 and a travel allowance of $750. In the second year, the stipend would increase by $3,000, but the travel allowance would remain the same.

• A selection committee for United Kingdom Visiting Fellows consisted of four distinguished United Kingdom biomedical scientists, including:

Walter Bodmer, Ph.D., F.R.S.
Director
Imperial Cancer Research

Sydney Brenner, Ph.D., F.R.S.
Head, Molecular Genetics Unit
Medical Research Council Laboratory of Molecular Biology
University of Cambridge School of Medicine

George Stark, Ph.D.
Chairman, Research Institute
The Cleveland Clinic

Sir David Weatherall, M.D., Ch.B., F.R.C.P., F.R.S.
Regis Professor of Medicine
University of Oxford

• A selection committee for Australian Visiting Fellows consisted of three distinguished Australian biomedical scientists, including:

Professor Emeritus Sir Gustov J. V. Nossal, A.C., C.B.E., Pres.A.A., F.R.S.
The Walther and Eliza Hall Institute of Medical Research

Professor Emeritus Donald Metcalf, A.C., M.D., F.A.A., F.R.S.
Assistant Director
The Walther and Eliza Hall Institute of Medical Research

Professor James Pittard, Ph.D. Yale, D.Sc. Melb, F.A.A.
Professor of Microbiology
University of Melbourne

• Each committee would invite 10 to 12 leading laboratories in the United Kingdom or Australia to nominate 1 or 2 candidates for the Markey Award. Nominees would be either at the postdoctoral or junior faculty level. The committee would review nominees and then hold one meeting to make final selections.

- The nominating institution would make a commitment to ensure placement of each Fellow upon their return to the United Kingdom or Australia.
- Each Fellow would obtain a commitment from a target United States institution, and, ideally, a preceptor within that institution.
- Funds for the Fellow would be paid to and administered by the targeted institution.
- Fellows were required to submit an annual progress report of their research accomplishments, along with a financial report from the targeted institution. The selection committee would review each Fellow's progress and provide overall surveillance of the program on a continuing basis.

EVALUATION OF THE VISITING FELLOWS PROGRAM

Because the Markey Visiting Fellows program was a postdoctoral award and because there was no comparison group, the committee decided not to conduct an evaluation of the outcomes of the Fellows program. We did interview as many Fellows as possible in order to gain an understanding of the impact of the postdoctoral fellowship on their research agenda and career pathway. It was much more difficult to locate and interview the Fellows, the majority of whom were living outside of the United States. A listing of the Markey Visiting Fellows and their locations at the time we contacted them to schedule an interview can be found in Appendix E of this report.

INTERVIEWS WITH MARKEY FELLOWS

A total of 29 Markey Visiting Fellows (23 men and 6 women) were interviewed between 1999 and 2004. When commenting on whether they felt independent prior to the start of the award, several U.K. Fellows mentioned that it is extremely difficult to complete a Ph.D. in the United Kingdom (a large percentage start and never finish), so actually finishing a dissertation almost guarantees that the individual is independent. More-over, the Fellows frequently noted that U.K. and Australian postdoctoral fellows were significantly younger than their U.S. counterparts because of the differences in the educational systems. As such, while they were intellectually very capable, there was a "ramping up" period when they first came to the United States where they needed to scramble in order to achieve the same level of productivity as their U.S. counterparts.

When I first joined the Markey program, I felt "out of depth"—but it was inspiring to meet these people [at the meetings] who had done such fantastic research.

The Markey raised my confidence level: being a young postdoctoral fellow in an established lab, and having changed fields totally, I needed all the confidence I could get.

When asked about their decisions to accept the Markey Fellowship, several Fellows noted that as they were already "the cream of the crop" they had other fellowship offers to study in the United States, but they selected the Markey Fellowship primarily for two reasons: 1) the award was to the individual, which meant they could change laboratories, if necessary and 2) the award had a more generous stipend than the others. One Fellow commented "this meant I had a nicer apartment, but it really didn't matter as I spent such little time there" (paraphrased). Another, by contrast, commented that the additional funds allowed him to add 6 months at the end of his fellowship period which allowed him to visit other U.S. laboratories, acquire additional techniques, and establish further collaborations before returning home.

I trotted around to various labs in the States, doing experiments in them . . . laying the groundwork for what I have gone on to do subsequently in my own lab. Had I not been paid generously by Markey, I probably would not have thought of spending my own money to do that.

Technology transfer was one of the goals of the Markey Visiting Fellows program. This was achieved when Fellows took new technologies with them when they returned to their home countries. The majority of the Fellows did return to their home countries at the completion of their fellowship. Of the 9 Fellows who continued working in the US, 5 are in academia, one is at a non-profit, and 3 are at biotechnology companies. The remainder have either returned to their home country, the United Kingdom or Australia, or are working in Europe or Asia—all at research institutes or in academia. Because of the lack of name-recognition outside the United States, only a small percentage of the Fellows commented that the Fellowship helped them find a job upon their return home. Those who did mention that the Award helped them find a job were mostly those who opted to stay in the United States. When queried as to what factors influenced a decision to accept a particular job offer, there were varied responses, including: dual career challenge, funding opportunities, wanting an urban setting (New York, London, or Tokyo), and a large number wanting to raise their families in their home countries.

It is more FUN doing science in Britain . . . you have more time to think; in the U.K. if you are good, you will be funded. Everyday life in the U.K. is less stressful than the U.S.

Australia has all the relatives, a better health care system, and generally a better environment for living.

These awards were initially for 2 years, with an optional third year. Many of the Fellows commented that unlike the Scholars, they did not feel the freedom to take on particularly riskier research because of the short duration of the award. At this point in the interview, when discussing the impact of the Visiting Fellow Award on their style of research, several individuals commented that the annual meetings had a significant impact on them. They referred frequently that "rubbing elbows" with the Markey Scholars and committee members was inspiring and one described it as a "boot-strapping" effect.

I don't think the structure of the award impacted my style, but definitely coming to the U.S. and staying for 5 years definitely impacted me in the sense that it made me familiar with how American science works. I better understand the mindset of U.S. scientists and the pressure to work in the lab all the time.

Working in the U.S. and being around the Scholars did impact me. I learned there was no one solution to a research question, and that multiple approaches with different tools have value.

Academic science is very competitive. People may not like the U.S. environment, but they need to see that these are the standards—this is the competition.

The Markey meetings exposed me to different areas of research. They created enthusiasm and fostered creative thinking. The fellowship gave me a more "expansive" view on research.

At the conclusion of their interviews, all but one Fellow noted that they felt they had met or exceeded, or were making significant progress toward meeting their career goals. The one person who felt he had not achieved his goals was doing far more clinical work than he wanted. All were appreciative of the opportunity to come to the United States and study, and felt that the program was an excellent postdoctoral award. Several mentioned that if a subsequent funder wanted to improve on the design of the award, it should consider extending the award term to include additional time to set up their laboratories when the Fellow returns to his or her home country.

Happiest two years of my life.

The personal side of the Markey Trust was very good. Other grant programs made you feel anonymous. I would recommend keeping the selection process rigorous. I take the European point of view—justified elitism. Don't give a little bit to everyone; give to very few and then the award will become a label of excellence.

I would like to thank the people who made the decisions for the opportunity. They gave me support to wander quite a long way from what I would imagine their support area [biomedicine] is.

The Markey was great because they didn't burden us with bureaucracy, and at the same time, what little they asked us to do was clearly assessed, seriously and appropriately.

6

Conclusions and Recommendations

There were two aspects of the Markey award that could account for differences between the Markey Scholars and comparison group members. One was the process used to select Markey Scholars. The other was the size, structure, and duration of the award itself. The committee could not differentiate the impacts of these two factors, but could evaluate the Markey Scholar award program generally. In doing so, the committee strongly concludes that the Markey Scholars program was successful.

Through a rigorous selection process, 113 Scholars were funded in seven cycles beginning in 1985 and continuing through 1991. Approximately 10 years after leaving the postdoctorate, these Scholars had made remarkable progress in their careers as research scientists. With only two exceptions, all Scholars had remained in biomedical research. Most of the Scholars had stayed as academic researchers in top-tier universities, and all had been tenured and promoted to associate or full professor. The Scholars who left academia for the biotechnology industry, research institutes, or NIH had equally responsible positions.

The Markey award, providing a generous stipend for up to seven years along with funding to establish a lab, enabled the Scholars to develop an independent research agenda, produce highly cited publications, and secure extramural funding. The data obtained for the committee's outcome measures show that Scholars were highly productive as measured by both the number of scholarly articles they produced and the number of citations these articles received. Scholars were also highly successful in obtaining extramural funding from NIH. Scholars in academia were awarded an average of 3.4 NIH grants during the 10-year interval that we surveyed or one grant every 3 years. More importantly, these Scholars received, on average, 2.0 R01 grants, or approximately one every 5 years.

The committee also concludes that the process used by the Markey Trust to nominate, screen, and select Scholars was effective in identifying biomedical researchers who would be able to rapidly advance to independence. In fact, many of the Scholars already considered their research to be independent at the time of the award.

The committee concludes that the annual Scholars Conference conducted by the Trust was an important component in the Scholars program. The Scholars Conference offered opportunities to network with other Scholars, members of the Scholar selection committee, and invited guests. In addition, it exposed Scholars to areas of biomedical science outside of their specialties.

Finally, while it did not have the impact of the Scholars program, the Visiting Fellows program made an important contribution in advancing biomedical research and in technology transfer.

Recommendation 1. Other funders, especially NIH, should consider creating awards that facilitate the transition from postdoctoral fellow to faculty status.

The committee recognizes that the transition from postdoctoral fellow to faculty status can be stressful. Moreover, very few funding programs provide career transition awards, although there has been recognition of the need for such programs for several years. A few years ago, the NRC Committee on Dimensions, Causes, and Implications of Recent Trends in the Careers of Life Scientists (National Research Council, 1998) recommended:

> Because of its concern for optimizing the creativity of young scientists and broadening the variety of scientific problems under study in the life sciences the committee recommends that public and private funding agencies establish "career-transition" grants for senior postdoctoral fellows. The intent is to identify the highest-quality scientists while they are still postdoctoral fellows and give them financial independence to begin new scientific projects of their own design in anticipation of their obtaining fully independent positions. The recommendation is based on the experience of the Lucille P. Markey Charitable Trust's Scholars in Biomedical Sciences Program.

In 1999, the NIH made the first of the K22 Career Transition Awards, designed to support an individual postdoctoral fellow in the transition to a faculty position. In the same year, the NIH instituted the K23 Mentored Patient-Oriented Research Career Development Award, for the development of the independent research scientist in the clinical area.

Recently, the NRC Committee on Bridges to Independence (National Research Council, 2005), headed by Thomas R. Cech recommended:

> NIH should establish a program to promote the conduct of innovative research by scientists transitioning into their first independent positions. These research grants, to replace the collection of K22 awards, would provide sufficient funding and resources for promising scientists to initiate an independent research program and allow for increased risk-taking during the final phase of their mentored postdoctoral training and during the initial phase of their independent research effort. The program should make 200 grants annually of $500,000 each, payable over 5 years.

This sentiment was echoed by the National Academies' Committee on Prospering in the Global Economy of the 21st Century (NAS/NAE/IOM, 2005b), which recommended:

> The federal government should establish a program to provide 200 new research grants each year at $500,000 each, payable over 5 years, to support work of the outstanding early-career researchers. The grants would be funded by federal agencies (NIH, NSF, DOD, DOE, and the National Aeronautics and Space Administration [NASA]) to underwrite new research opportunities at universities and government agencies.

The committee strongly endorses these recommendations and commends the National Institutes of Health for developing the new Pathway to Independence awards (National Institutes of Health, 2006b) that will fund between 150 and 200 awards that will foster the early independence of new investigators. The Pathway to Independence award was made partially in response to the recommendations of the *Bridges to Independence* committee.

Recommendation 2. Other funders of biomedical researchers should consider adopting the template developed by the Markey Trust.

The Markey Scholars Award provided a template that can be used by philanthropic and governmental funders (especially the NIH) to identify and fund biomedical scientists at this important time in their careers. The committee recommends that any future funders of career transitions awards give careful consideration to this template since it can enable funders to (1) identify postdoctoral fellows who believe that they are independent or nearly independent in their research agenda, (2) provide funding not only for salaries but also for laboratory equipment, supplies, and staff, and (3) monitor awardees to ensure that they establish independent research careers in a timely manner. The committee urges funders to make certain that institutions making nominations ensure that female and minority nominees are fully included in all aspects of the nomination process. Moreover, the committee recommends that future funders incorporate annual meetings modeled after the Markey Scholars Conference to enable awardees to benefit from networking. Finally, both the Scholars and comparison group members offered several innovative suggestions for features that went beyond the Markey template and might enhance the funding of biomedical scientists. The committee recommends that any future funders consider these suggestions as part of the funding process.

Recommendation 3. The committee recommends funding to foster the international exchange of biomedical scientists for research and training.

The committee recommends that funders establish mechanisms to bring foreign biomedical scientists to laboratories in the United States for intensive research and training and to fund research and training opportunities for U.S. biomedical scientists abroad. The increasing globalization of science and engineering, especially biomedical science, was ably demonstrated by a 2005 report from the National Academies' Committee on Science, Engineering, and Public Policy report (NAS/NAE/IOM, 2005a). The report stated:

> The United States has benefited from the inflow of talented students and scholars. Migrants to the United States tend to be more educated than the average person in the sending country, and the proportion of highly educated people who emigrate is high. Many people believe that emigration of the technically skilled—"brain drain"—is detrimental to the country of origin. Some effects on the sending country described by scholars are higher domestic wages, lost economies of scale, reduction in specialized skills, and slower resource reallocation to learning-intensive sectors. Others argue that the migration of scholars benefits both sending and receiving countries, providing access to leading research and training not available in the home country and creating transnational bridges to cutting-edge research. In general, the concept of "brain drain" may be too simplistic inasmuch as it ignores many benefits of emigration, including remittances, international collaborations, the return of skilled

scientists and engineers, diaspora-facilitated international business, and a general investment in skills caused by the prospect of emigration. Some researchers argue that, as the R&D enterprise becomes more global, "brain drain" should be recast as "brain circulation" and include the broader topics of the international circulation of thinkers, knowledge workers, and rights to knowledge. Such a discussion would include issues of local resources; many countries lack the educational and technical infrastructure to support advanced education, so aspiring scientists and engineers have little choice but to seek at least part of their training abroad, and in many instances such travel is encouraged by governments.

Recommendation 4. Any funders of biomedical researchers should incorporate a prospective, data-driven monitoring and evaluation system as part of the program.

The committee strongly believes that a data-driven, prospective evaluation should be fully integrated into any new funding initiative. The committee recommends that funders undertake (at least) annual monitoring of awardee activities for several years. Data generated from monitoring should be used to target appropriate candidates and tailor funding to meet changing needs. The committee notes that many philanthropic and public funders rigorously monitor and evaluate the outcomes of awardees and use these assessments to guide future funding strategies (National Research Council, 2006).

Recommendation 5. The biotechnology industry and the government are making important contributions to the biomedical research agenda and should not be excluded from transitional funding mechanisms.

The committee recognizes that the biotechnology industry and government are increasingly attractive destinations for biomedical researchers. It recommends that current and future funders of biomedical scientists continue support for those who transition to these destinations outside of academia.

In conclusion, the committee believes that the Markey Scholars Awards program is a useful model for funding biomedical researchers that should be considered by other funders. The committee recognizes that 5 to 7 years of support at a critical time of development, with funding more flexible than at many other programs, has produced many successful scientists. The Burroughs Wellcome Fund has developed the Career Award

Program in the Biomedical Sciences (CABS), which is modeled after the Markey Scholar Awards program (National Research Council, 2006). In addition, the American Heart Association's Fellow-to-Faculty Award and the National Multiple Sclerosis Society Career Transition Fellowships fund this important time of career transition. The committee also endorses new programs, such as NIH's Pioneer Award, that foster independent research agendas for biomedical scientists later in their careers.

References

Association of American Medical Colleges. 1988. Medical Student Graduation Question-naire, 1988: Summary Report for all Schools. Available at www.aamc.org/data/gq/allschoolsreports/1988.pdf.

Auerbach, Ann Hagedorn. 1994. *Wild Ride: The Rise and Fall of Calumet Farm, Inc., America's Premier Racing Dynasty*. New York: Henry Holt and Company.

Burroughs Wellcome Fund and Howard Hughes Medical Institute. 2004. *Making the Right Moves: A Practical Guide to Scientific Management for Postdocs and New Faculty.*

Dickason, John H. and Duncan Neuhauser. 2000. *Closing a Foundation: The Lucille P. Markey Charitable Trust*. Washington, DC: Council on Foundations.

Fichtner, Margaret. 1990. "Mrs. Markey's Money: She Willed Her Wealth to Science, Trust Decides Who Gets it." Miami Herald. December 2.

Ginsberg, Eli and Anna B. Dutka. 1989. *The Financing of Biomedical Research*. Baltimore, MD: The Johns Hopkins University Press.

Lucille P. Markey Charitable Trust. 1984. *Lucille P. Markey Scholar Awards in Biomedical Science, 1984*. Miami, FL: Lucille P. Markey Charitable Trust.

Lucille P. Markey Charitable Trust. 1988. *Report 1983-1988*. Miami, FL: Lucille P. Markey Charitable Trust.

Lucille P. Markey Charitable Trust. 1991. *Program Information and Guidelines 1991*. Miami, FL: Lucille P. Markey Charitable Trust.

Lucille P. Markey Charitable Trust. 1995. *1995 Scholars Conference and Symposium on General Organizational Programs*. Chicago, Ill.: Lucille P. Markey Charitable Trust.

Lucille P. Markey Charitable Trust. 1996. *Final Report 1983-1996*. Miami, FL: Lucille P. Markey Charitable Trust.

Lucille P. Markey Charitable Trust Records. 1981-(1983-1966)-1998. Sleepy Hollow, NY: Rockefeller Archive Center.

National Academy of Sciences, National Academy of Engineering, and Institute of Medicine (NAS/NAE/IOM). 2005a. *Policy Implications of International Graduate Students and Post-doctoral Scholars in the United States*. Washington, DC: The National Academies Press.

NAS/NAE/IOM. 2005b. *Rising Above the Gathering Storm: Energizing and Employing America for a Brighter Economic Future*. Washington, DC: The National Academies Press.

National Institutes of Health (NIH). 2001. Average Size of NIH Traditional Research Project (R01) Awards. Available at http://grants1.nih.gov/grants/award/research/avgr01fy6801.htm.

NIH. 2003. NIH Competing Career Development Applications–Success Rates Fiscal Years 1970–2003. By Funding Mechanism (Activity). Available at http://grants1.nih.gov/grants/award/training/comrcp7003.htm.

NIH. 2006a. Research Grants Award Data. Available at http://grants1.nih.gov/grants/award/resgr.htm.

NIH. 2006b. NIH Announces Programs to Foster the Independence of New Investigators. Available at http://grants.nih.gov/grants/new_investigators/index.htm.

National Research Council (NRC). 1995. *Research Doctorate Programs in the United States: Continuity and Change.* Washington, DC: National Academy Press.

NRC. 1998. *Trends in the Early Careers of Life Scientists.* Washington, DC: National Academy Press.

NRC. 2005. *Bridges to Independence: Fostering the Independence of New Investigators in Biomedical Research.* Washington, DC: The National Academies Press.

NRC. 2006. *Enhancing Philanthropy's Support of Biomedical Scientists: Proceedings of a Workshop on Methodology.* Washington, DC: The National Academies Press.

National Science Foundation, Division of Science Resources Studies. 1997. *Science and Engineering Doctorates Awards: 1996: Detailed Statistical Tables.* NSF 97-329, by Susan T. Hill. Arlington, VA: National Science Foundation.

Nicklin, Julie L. 1997. "Markey Trust, Having Given $500-Million, Will Close This Year." The Chronicle of Higher Education. February 28.

Spradley, James P. 1983. *The Ethnographic Interview.* New York: Holt, Rinehart, & Winston.

Appendixes

Appendix A

Committee Members
Biographical Information

Enriqueta Bond, Ph.D., is President of the Burroughs-Wellcome Fund. She is a former Executive Director of the Institute of Medicine of which she is also a member. Her research interests include genetics, molecular biology, and science policy. She has served on the IOM's Board on Health Sciences Policy and on the Committee to Study Incentives for Resource Sharing in the Biomedical Sciences. She holds a Ph.D. in biology.

William T. Butler, M.D., is Chancellor Emeritus of Baylor College of Medicine where he is also Professor of Internal Medicine and Professor of Immunology. He served as the College's President and Chief Executive Officer from 1979 to 1996. Before joining the Baylor faculty in 1966, Dr. Butler served as the chief clinical associate at the National Institute of Allergy and Infectious Diseases at the NIH. He served on the boards of Browning-Ferris Industries, C. R. Bard, Inc., and Lyondell Chemical, where he is Chairman of the Board. Dr. Butler has done extensive research on the effects of corticosteroids and other drugs on the immune system and the mechanism of rejection of organ transplants. Dr. Butler holds an M.D. (1958) from Western Reserve University and a B.A. (1954) from Oberlin College. Dr. Butler is a member of the Institute of Medicine.

Elaine K. Gallin, Ph.D., is the Program Director for Medical Research at The Doris Duke Charitable Foundation. Dr. Gallin's research involves the characterization of ion transport mechanisms in macrophages, leukocyte-endothelial cell interactions, and the effects of ionizing radiation of leukocyte function and vascular integrity. She received her B.S. from

75

Cornell University, her M.S. from Hunter College, and her Ph.D. from City University, New York. She has held positions at the Uniformed Services University, Georgetown University Medical School, was a Congressional Fellow on the Public Policy Committee, and is a member of the Physiology Study Section at NIH.

Mary-Lou Pardue, Ph.D., is the Boris Magasanik Professor of Biology at the Massachusetts Institute of Technology and a member of the National Academy of Sciences. As a geneticist and cell biologist, she has studied eukaryotic chromosomes with emphasis on sequences involved in the structure and function of chromosomes as organelles. She served as president of both the Genetics Society of America and the American Society for Cell Biology and was Chair of the Institute of Medicine Committee on Understanding of Biology of Sex and Gender Difference. She received a Ph.D. from Yale University in 1970.

Georgine Pion, Ph.D., is Research Associate Professor of Psychology and Human Development and Senior Fellow with the Vanderbilt Institute for Public Policy Studies at Vanderbilt University. She received her Ph.D. in social-environmental psychology from Claremont Graduate School in 1980 and did postdoctoral research training in the Division of Methodology and Evaluation Research at Northwestern University. She has served on committees involved in the evaluation of research and health professional training programs and gender differences in the career development of scientists for the National Research Council, the National Science Foundation, and the National Institute of Mental Health. Currently, she is involved in directing an evaluation of the neuroscience peer review process at the NIH, evaluating the outcomes of new instructional strategies in biomedical engineering education, and assessing the outcomes of postdoctoral research training programs sponsored by the Burroughs Wellcome Fund and other foundations. She is an Associate of the National Academy of Sciences

Lloyd Hollingsworth Smith, M.D., is Professor Emeritus of Medicine and a former Associate Dean of the School of Medicine at the University of California, San Francisco. His areas of expertise include biochemistry, endocrinology and metabolism, internal medicine, and medical genetics. His interests and capabilities also include medical center administration, medical education, training of investigators, and medical research policy. Dr. Smith holds an M.D. (1948) from Harvard Medical School and a B.A. (1944) from Washington & Lee University. Dr. Smith is a past member of the Board of Overseers of Harvard University. He is a member of the Institute of Medicine. He has previously served on the Committee to Study

Strategies to Strengthen the Scientific Excellence of the NIH Intramural Research Program.

Lee Sechrest, Ph.D., is Professor of Psychology at the University of Arizona. His primary interest is in development and improvement of methods for research and data analysis, particularly for research in field settings. He is also involved in program evaluation. Substantive areas include health and mental health services, clinical psychology, and personality. Additional areas of expertise include research methodology, measurement, program evaluation, quality assurance in service delivery, and quality of scientific information. He is interested and involved in matters having to do with the development of psychology as a responsible, science-based profession. Before coming to Arizona, he held faculty positions in Pennsylvania State University, Northwestern University, Florida State University, and the University of Michigan. He received his Ph.D. from the Ohio State University. Dr. Sechrest has served on five NRC study committees, including the Panel to Study Gender Differences in the Career Outcomes of Science and Engineering Ph.D.s.

Virginia Weldon, M.D., is retired Senior Vice President for Public Policy with the Monsanto Company. In this position she identified public policy issues affecting the company and planned for and orchestrated Monsanto's approach to these issues. Prior to joining Monsanto in 1989, Dr. Weldon was Professor of Pediatrics and Associate Vice Chancellor for Medical Affairs at the Washington University School of Medicine. Dr. Weldon is on the Board of Directors of G.D. Searle & Company, The NutraSweet Company, and the Monsanto Fund. She holds an M.D. (1962) from the University of Buffalo and an A.B. (1957) from Smith College. She is a member of the Institute of Medicine and serves on the Report Review Committee of the National Research Council and Institute of Medicine.

James Wyngaarden, M.D., is Professor Emeritus at Duke University. At Duke, Dr. Wyngaarden served as Associate Vice Chancellor for Health Affairs, Chief of Staff and Physician-in-Chief at Duke University Hospital, and Frederic M. Hanes Professor and Chairman, Department of Medicine at the Duke University School of Medicine. From 1982 to 1989, Dr. Wyngaarden was Director, U.S. National Institutes of Health, and from 1989 to 1990 was Associate Director for Life Sciences, White House Office of Science and Technology Policy. Dr. Wyngaarden holds an M.D. (1948) from the University of Michigan Medical School. He is a member of the National Academy of Sciences and the Institute of Medicine and is a former Foreign Secretary of the NAS and IOM.

Appendix B

History of the Markey Trust[1]

L ucille P. Markey executed her will creating the Lucille P. Markey Charitable Trust in 1975. Mrs. Markey's wealth, which later endowed the Trust, was derived from the family of her first husband, Warren Wright. In 1888, with an initial investment of $3,500, Warren's father, William Wright, founded the Calumet Baking Powder Company, which he built over the ensuing decades into the leading company in the industry. In the late 1920s, Warren sold Calumet to Postum (later General Foods) for about $32 million. This fortune, along with Calumet Farms, purchased by the elder Wright in 1924, was the foundation of the Wrights' wealth, the bulk of which passed to Warren. When Warren Wright died in 1950, his estate was valued at approximately $20 million, about half of which was in securities and a quarter in oil and gas interests in seven states that would appreciate significantly in later years (Auerbach, 1994).

One of the valuable Wright-owned oil fields was the Waddell Ranch located outside of Odessa, Texas. Under typical oil lease arrangements, the lessor—in this case Gulf Oil Company—paid all costs and received seven-eighths of the proceeds, while the property owner received one-eighth. In 1925, Gulf Oil leased the Waddell Ranch for 50 years, an unusual arrangement as most oil leases were for perpetuity or for as long as the

---

[1]The History of the Markey Trust is largely a duplicate of the same section that appeared in Funding Biomedical Research Programs: Contributions of the Markey Trust. The committee wants each of the five reports produced in this evaluation to exist independently; consequently some sections are repeated in each report.

land is productive. In 1975, following the oil embargo and consequent rapid increase in oil prices, the leases expired. Through a series of court cases, Gulf fought to have the leases extended at the old 1925 rate, but eventually the Wright heirs and the other Waddell Ranch owners were victorious and the income from the new leases, which were then part of Mrs. Markey's estate, increased dramatically. Prior to his death, Warren Wright had amply addressed the needs of his children through a trust arrangement. Lucille Wright, who subsequently married Eugene Markey, realized that her estate would go either to charity or taxes. Mrs. Markey concluded that she was not interested in leaving her money to charity as broadly defined, but rather to something that would be immediate and specific (Auerbach, 1994).

Mrs. Markey's decision to leave her estate to medical research evolved slowly. Her illnesses and those of Gene Markey stimulated her interest in research that could impact human health. Realizing that health research is a broad field, Mrs. Markey asked Louis Hector, her attorney, to explore whether something more specific could be identified to guide the work of the charity. Hector visited the Robert Wood Johnson Foundation, which was established in 1972 as a national philanthropy devoted to improving the health and health care of all Americans, and the Rockefeller University, which focuses on medical research, to learn more of their activities. After hearing of the work of both institutions, Mrs. Markey concluded that the clinical aspects of health care were covered by other institutions, and that her estate should be dedicated to the promotion of biomedical research. Because of this decision the term "basic medical research" was inserted into her will.

> It took her quite a while to wrap her mind around the idea of basic medical research," says Hector, "but once she did, that was it. The money, she decided, should go for square-one stuff, to solve the most elemental and perplexing puzzles. (Fichtner, 1990).

The mission of the Markey Trust, thus was "For the purposes of supporting and encouraging basic medical research" (Lucille P. Markey Charitable Trust, 1996).

Although she had not previously been a generous benefactor, Mrs. Markey began to respond to solicitations from a variety of local institutions. The following anecdote reveals how her giving began with the University of Kentucky:

> When Dr. Roach first approached Lucille Markey in the late 1970s for a contribution toward the construction of a cancer center on the campus

of the University of Kentucky, she said graciously, "Of course, Ben, we'll
help. We'll give you $1,000." In response, Gene Markey chimed in, "Dear,
he doesn't want a thousand dollars, he wants a million." The next morn-
ing Mrs. Markey called Dr. Roach and said, "We're going to give you one
million in cash for your center." (Auerbach, 1994:95-96).

She subsequently gave a number of gifts totaling $5.25 million to
the Ephraim McDowell Research Foundation to build a cancer center
at the University of Kentucky. In 1984 and 1985, the Markey Trust gave
nearly $8.1 million to the University of Kentucky to continue programs
Mrs. Markey had initiated before her death (Lucille P. Markey Charitable
Trust, 1996).

In addition to settling on a substantive focus for her Trust, Mrs. Markey
also determined that she did not want to create a permanent foundation
that might change or drift away from her own mission. Rather, she wanted
to disperse her estate quickly so that the work of the Trust would not
change over time, particularly as the Trustees changed. Louis J. Hector,
who became chairman of the Trust, once told *The Chronicle of Higher Education* that when he and Mrs. Markey were working out the details of the
Trust, the heiress told him, "I want the money out there doing a job, and
I think what the trustees ought to do is spend it in a reasonable amount
of time and then shut down" (Nicklin, 1997).

Mrs. Markey elected to limit the term of the Trust to 15 years and
the number of trustees to five. Her decision was based on four guiding
principles (Dickason and Neuhauser, 2000:2):

1. She felt it was important to apply as much money as possible to
achieving the Trust's purpose in as short a time as possible.

2. She wanted to know who would be involved in the management
of the assets and distribution of her largess. She named five trustees, all
of whom she knew well. Four of them were alive at her death and three
continued to serve throughout the life of the Trust.

3. She wanted her money applied to grants, not to support a permanent bureaucracy.

4. She believed that the purpose and goals of any foundation could
become obsolete over time; a time limit could help to prevent such
obsolescence.

When Mrs. Markey died on July 24, 1982, the Lucille P. Markey Charitable Trust was incorporated as a Florida nonprofit organization with
501(c) (3) status. The initial meeting of the Board of Trustees occurred in
October 1983, and the Trust's Miami office opened January 1, 1984. The
trust completed all activities on June 15, 1997.

Four trustees attended the initial 1983 meeting (Dickason and Neuhauser, 2000):

1. Laurette Heraty, who had served Mrs. Markey and her first husband, Warren Wright, in their Chicago office as a secretary since 1937. She retired from the board in 1989.
2. Louis Hector, who was Mrs. Markey's attorney and drafted her will. He served as a trustee of the University of Miami, Rockefeller University, and the Lincoln Center and is a member of the American Academy of Arts and Sciences.
3. William Sutter, an attorney and expert in oil and gas leasing issues, who worked for Mr. Wright and Mrs. Markey from his Chicago office in the law firm of Hopkins and Sutter.
4. Margaret Glass of Lexington, Kentucky, who worked so closely with Mrs. Markey over the years that she was seen as an effective custodian and interpreter of her wishes.

Two additional trustees were named during the life of the Trust:

1. George Shinn, a financial expert (elected to fill the position left vacant by the death in 1980 of Gene Markey) was president of Merrill Lynch & Co., CEO of First Boston Corporation, and a member of the Board of Governors of the New York Stock Exchange.
2. Robert Glaser, a physician with experience in both academic medicine and philanthropy (elected in 1989 following the retirement of Laurette Heraty), was the Trust's Director of Medical Sciences from 1984 until 1989. He was past president of the Henry J. Kaiser Family Foundation and dean of the University of Colorado Medical School and Stanford University School of Medicine.

The structure and the function of the Markey Trust were guided from its inception by Louis Hector's vision of supporting and encouraging basic medical research. This vision was consistent and unwavering throughout the duration of the trust and guided the selection of grantees, advisers, reviewers, and funding mechanisms.

Dr. Glaser also played a critical role in guiding the implementation of the Markey Trust programs. In 1984, he was asked to become the director of medical sciences for the Trust. Some of his initial recommendations to the Trust included the idea of supporting basic (as opposed to targeted) research. "Medicine was going through an exciting period," Glaser recalled. "There were new fields like structural biology and developmental biology coming along and with substantial resources such as the Trust enjoyed, they could do a very important thing by offering support that was flexible to people and/or programs over a period of time" (Glaser, 2002). Dr. Glaser also recommended that the Trust provide enough support to bright young people to allow them protected time to establish their research careers. His expertise and vision were to become the major force in the foundation.

The Trust began distributing funds in 1984 to institutions that Mrs. Markey had supported during her lifetime. At the same time, the Trust began to plan a long-term strategy for its programs. In 1984, the Trust held a series of three "think tank" meetings with distinguished biomedical researchers in California, New York, and London. These sessions produced a number of recommendations, the most important of which was the idea of long-term financial support for postdoctoral fellows and young faculty members. In 1984 the Trust announced the creation of the Markey Scholars Awards in Biomedical Sciences, which became the Trust's best-known program. The initial cohort of Markey Scholars was appointed in February 1985. In the fall of 1985, the initial Research Program Grants were awarded. Later, in 1988, the Trust began making what would later be classified as General Organizational Grants. Each of these award mechanisms is discussed in greater detail later.

In 1985, most Trust activity ceased because of complicated litigation involving the pricing of natural gas. The litigation involved the Federal Energy Regulatory Commission, the California Public Service Commission, and a number of major oil and gas companies. The case was eventually settled in Texas courts. However, during the two years of court proceedings, the Trust funded no new research grants and was able to continue funding only for the Markey Scholars program and for a few small miscellaneous and related grants. During this hiatus, the Trustees continued to receive new grant proposals and conducted selected site visits. Moreover, the value of the Markey Estate and Trust grew substantially, benefiting from investment income as well as the continued oil and gas income. In the fall of 1987 the litigation was resolved, and the Trust resumed awarding Research Program Grants. During its 15-year lifetime, the Markey Trust gave a total of $507,151,000 to basic medical research and research training. Administrative costs amounted to $29,087,000, or approximately 5 percent of the total Trust. A recent study by the Urban Institute indicates that foundations of similar size and scope have average operating and administrative expenses of about 8 percent (Boris, et. al., 2005). Additional expenses included $10,529,000 for direct investment costs and mineral depletion costs. The total value of the Trust was $549,520,000, which included $149,565,000 in investment income (Dickason and Neuhauser, 2000).

Appendix C

Lucille P. Markey
Charitable Trust Programs

The Markey Trust made awards in the three main stages of a biomedical research career in which "supporting and encouraging basic medical research" can occur.

1. General Organizational Grants were directed to improve the education and training of both Ph.D.s and M.D.s planning careers in basic clinical research and research in molecular medicine.

2. Markey Scholars and Fellows Awards identified and supported outstanding younger researchers in the biomedical sciences, providing them with long-term financial assistance early in their careers.

3. Research Program Grants provided funding opportunities for established scientists with proven records of excellence in biomedical research.

A few grants that fell outside the above categories were put into a miscellaneous category. The distribution of funding is shown in Figure C-1. This Appendix describes the General Organizational Grants program, Research Program Grants, and miscellaneous awards.

GENERAL ORGANIZATIONAL GRANTS

Almost at its inception, The Markey Trust had become cognizant of a growing gap between biomedical research and clinical application. In 1989, input was sought from a number of biomedical scientists on directions for Trust funding during its remaining term. They advised that there

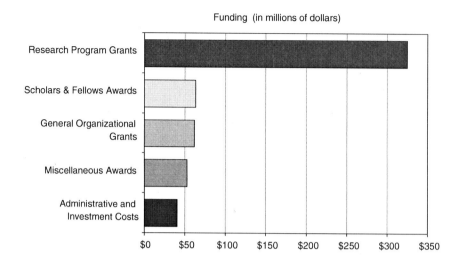

FIGURE C-1 Distribution of Markey funding across programs and grant making. SOURCE: Lucille P. Markey Charitable Trust, 1996.

was general concern in medical schools about the "bed-bench gap" and that plans were emerging in many universities to develop new curricula and teaching techniques to close the gap between laboratory research and research based on clinical observation.

The Markey Trust indicated that it would be responsive to proposals to address the development of training programs designed to bridge the "bed-bench" gap. The trustees received a number of proposals that fell into two categories: those that provided significant opportunities for M.D.s to engage in basic research during and immediately following medical school and residency and those that provided significant clinical exposure for Ph.D.s while they were predoctoral or postdoctoral students. The first of these awards, classified as General Organizational Grants, was made in 1992. These grants were designed to close the widening gap between rapid advances in our understanding of biological process and the translation of that knowledge into techniques for preventing diseases (Lucille P. Markey Charitable Trust, 1995).

General Organizational Grant programs were funded for approximately five years, although due to the flexibility of the Markey grants, many grant recipients were able to extend the grant's duration. Because of the limited term of the Trust, General Organizational Grants could not be renewed. Between 1988 and 1995, 22 General Organizational Grants amounting to $62,121,700 were awarded. The average amount awarded was about $2.8 million, but award amounts ranged from $50,000 to $13,750,000.

RESEARCH PROGRAM GRANTS

The largest Markey awards in terms of funding amount and number of projects were the Research Program Grants. These grants were designed to enable investigators to address important issues in the biomedical sciences by developing new approaches or expanding continuing approaches to the study of basic biomedical fields.

Research Program Grants were made to institutions with a major commitment to the life sciences to assist in the establishment, reorganization, or expansion of significant biomedical research programs or centers. The grants usually involved funding for the recruitment of new faculty, pre- and postdoctoral support, completion or renovation of laboratory space, purchase of new equipment, and additional technical assistance (Lucille P. Markey Charitable Trust, 1988). Moreover, Research Program Grants were intended to fund research that, generally, would not be funded by the National Institutes of Health.

Generally, grants were awarded for five years. Because of the limited term of the Trust, awardees were advised that the grants were not renewable. The Trust made 92 Research Program Grants between the years of 1986 and 1995 amounting to over $316,248,175. In 1996 and 1997 the Trust made 18 supplementary awards of $500,000 each, bring the total awarded funding of Research Program Grants to $325,248,175.

MISCELLANEOUS AWARDS

During its tenure, the Markey Trust made a number of awards that did not fit into the three major award categories. These awards continued support made by Mrs. Markey during her lifetime, funded endowed chairs, provided scholarships to biomedical researchers, and funded related research support. These award programs, totaling $53,606,232, are listed below.

Lucille P. Markey Basic Medical Research Funds

To memorialize the Trust's support for the training of biomedical scientists, endowments totaling $14,000,000 were made to seven institutions. These institutions established permanent endowments known as the

Lucille P. Markey Basic Medical Research Funds to provide support for promising predoctoral and postdoctoral fellows and junior faculty.[1]

Markey Predoctoral Fellows

In its early years the Trust provided $9,400,000 to 15 academic institutions to assist predoctoral students in biomedical science programs. These graduate students were known as Markey Fellows.

Other Grants for Career Development

The Trust provided $3,030,000 to six research institutes to fund summer seminars and short courses for potential scientists in basic medical research.[2]

Continuation of Programs Initiated by Mrs. Markey

These awards were made in 1984 and 1985 to the University of Kentucky and University of Miami and totaled $8,700,000.

Endowed Chairs

Between 1985 and 1996, the Markey Trust provided $11,500,000 to fund endowed chairs.[3]

Research Support and Related Grants

Between 1985 and 1997, the Trust provided $6,976,232 to fund 56 miscellaneous grants to support smaller research projects and to encourage or facilitate basic medical research.

---

[1]These seven institutions were: Harvard University, Johns Hopkins University, Rockefeller University, Stanford University, University of California, San Francisco, University of Michigan, and University of Texas Southwestern Medical Center.

[2]These include: Cold Spring Harbor Laboratory, Jackson Laboratory, Marine Biology Laboratory, Mount Desert Island Biological Laboratory, Vassar College, and Life Sciences Research Foundation.

[3]The endowed chairs were: Rockefeller University, Henry G. Kunkel Professor; University of Kentucky, Warren Wright, Sr.-Lucille Wright Markey Chair, Gluck Equine Research Center; University of Kentucky, Lucille P. Markey Chair in Oncology Research; University of Kentucky, Warren Wright, Sr.-Lucille Wright Markey Chair, Gluck Equine Research Center (supplement); University of Miami, Markey Professorship in Biochemistry and Molecular Biology; Washington University in St. Louis, Markey Professorship in Basic Biomedical or Basic Biological Sciences; and Yale University, Lucille P. Markey Professorship in Biomedical Sciences.

Appendix D

Markey Scholar Awards in Biomedical Sciences

James M. Anderson, M.D., Ph.D.
Professor
Yale University School of Medicine
New Haven, CT

Paul H. Axelsen, M.D.
Associate Professor
University of Pennsylvania
Philadelphia, PA

Jay M. Baraban, M.D., Ph.D.
Associate Professor
Johns Hopkins University
Baltimore, MD

Cornelia Bargmann, Ph.D.
Professor and Associate Investigator
University of California, San Francisco/HHMI
San Francisco, CA

Margaret H. Baron, M.D., Ph.D.
Associate Professor
The Mount Siani School of Medicine
New York, NY

Joseph M. Beechem, M.D., Ph.D.
Director of Biosciences
Molecular Probes
Eugene, OR

Howard Benjamin, Ph.D.
Vice President, Discovery Research
Praecus Pharmaceuticals, Inc.
Cambridge, MA

Mark S. Braiman, Ph.D.
Professor
Syracuse University
Syracuse, NY

Stephen J. Brandt, M.D.
Associate Professor
Vanderbilt University
Nashville, TN

Patrick Brown, M.D., Ph.D.
Associate Professor and Investigator
Stanford University/HHMI
Stanford, CA

Michael L. Cleary, M.D.
Associate Professor
Stanford University
Stanford, CA

John A. Cooper, M.D., Ph.D.
Professor
Washington University School of Medicine
St. Louis, MO

Stephen T. Crews, Ph.D.
Associate Professor
University of North Carolina, Chapel Hill
Chapel Hill, NC

Frederick R. Cross, M.D., Ph.D.
Professor and Head of Laboratory
The Rockefeller University
New York, NY

Martha S. Cyert, Ph.D.
Associate Professor
Stanford University
Stanford, CA

Alan D. D'Andrea, M.D.
Professor
Dana-Farber Cancer Institute
Boston, MA

Seth A. Darst, Ph.D.
Professor and Head of Laboratory
The Rockefeller University
New York, NY

Laura I. Davis, Ph.D.
Affiliate
Massachusetts Institute of Technology
Cambridge, MA

Michael A. Davitz, M.D., J.D.
Associate
White & Case
New York, NY

Titia de Lange, Ph.D.
Professor and Head of Laboratory
The Rockefeller University
New York, NY

Raymond J. Deshaies, Ph.D.
Associate Professor and Investigator
California Institute of Technology/HHMI
Pasadena, CA

Stephen DiNardo, Ph.D.
Professor
University of Pennsylvania School of Medicine
Philadelphia, PA

Jennifer A. Doudna, Ph.D.
Professor and Investigator
Yale University School of Medicine/HHMI
New Haven, CT

Allison Doupe, M.D., Ph.D.
Professor
University of California, San Francisco
San Francisco, CA

William G. Dunphy, Ph.D.
Associate Professor and Assistant In
California Institute of Technology/HHMI
Pasadena, CA

Geoffrey M. Duyk, M.D., Ph.D.
Director
Exelixis Pharmaceuticals
Cambridge, MA

Bruce A. Edgar, Ph.D.
Member
Fred Hutchinson Cancer Research Institute
Seattle, WA

Thomas E. Ellenberger, D.V.M., Ph.D.
Professor
Harvard Medical School
Boston, MA

Joanne N. Engel, M.D., Ph.D.
Associate Professor
University of California, San Francisco
San Francisco, CA

James J. Figge, M.D.
Director, Thyroid Cancer Program
St. Peter's Hospital
Albany, NY

Stephen H. Friend, M.D., Ph.D.
President
Rosetta Pharmaceuticals
Kirkland, WA

Robert S. Fuller, Ph.D.
Associate Professor
University of Michigan
Ann Arbor, MI

Abram Gabriel, M.D.
Associate Professor
Rutgers University
Piscataway, NJ

Jeff Gelles, Ph.D.
Professor
Brandeis University
Waltham, MA

Alfred L. George, Jr., M.D.
Professor
Vanderbilt University
Nashville, TN

Christopher K. Glass, M.D., Ph.D.
Professor
University of California, San Diego
San Diego, CA

Alan L. Goldin, M.D., Ph.D.
Professor
University of California, Irvine
Irvine, CA

Adrian Goldman, Ph.D.
Professor
University of Turku
Turku, Finland

Eric D. Green, M.D., Ph.D.
Scientific Director, NHGRI
National Institutes of Health
Bethesda, MD

Alan Davis Grossman, Ph.D.
Associate Professor
Massachusetts Institute of Technology
Cambridge, MA

Kathleen B. Hall, Ph.D.
Associate Professor
Washington University School of Medicine
St. Louis, MO

Min Han, Ph.D.
Associate Professor and Investigator
University of Colorado, Boulder/HHMI
Boulder, CO

Jeffrey D. Hardin, Ph.D.
Professor
University of Wisconsin
Madison, WA

Wendy Lynn Havran, Ph.D.
Associate Professor
The Scripps Research Institute
La Jolla, CA

Gail E. Hermann, M.D., Ph.D.
Professor
Ohio State University
Columbus, OH

Daniel Herschlag, Ph.D.
Professor
Stanford University
Stanford, CA

Joachim J. Herz, M.D.
Associate Professor
University of Texas Southwestern Medical Center
Dallas, TX

David M. Hockenbery, M.D.
Member
Fred Hutchinson Cancer Research Institute
Seattle, WA

Merl F. Hoekstra, Ph.D.
Vice President
Epoch Biosciences
Monroe, WA

Anthony Hyman, Ph.D.
Director
Director, Max Planck Institute of Molecular Cell Biology and Genetics
Dresden, Germany

Tyler E. Jacks, Ph.D.
Professor and Investigator
Massachusetts Institute of Technology/HHMI
Cambridge, MA

Daniel G. Jay, Ph.D.
Associate Professor
Tufts University
Cambridge, MA

James T. Kadonaga, Ph.D.
Professor
University of California, San Diego
San Diego, CA

Chris A. Kaiser, Ph.D.
Professor
Massachusetts Institute of Technology
Cambridge, MA

Lawrence C. Katz, Ph.D.
Professor and Investigator
Duke University Medical Center/HHMI
Durham, NC

Carolyn J. Kelly, M.D.
Associate Professor
University of California, San Diego
San Diego, CA

Daniel P. Kelly, M.D.
Professor
Washington University School of Medicine
St. Louis, MO

Stuart K. Kim, Ph.D.
Professor
Stanford University Medical School
Stanford, CA

David M. Kingsley, Ph.D.
Associate Professor and Investigator
Stanford University Medical School/HHMI
Stanford, CA

M. Magda Konarska, Ph.D.
Associate Professor and Head of Laboratory
The Rockefeller University
New York, NY

Ron Rieger Kopito, Ph.D.
Professor
Stanford University
Stanford, CA

Douglas E. Koshland, Ph.D.
Member and Investigator
Carnegie Institution of Washington/HHMI
Baltimore, M.D

Mark A. Krasnow, M.D., Ph.D.
Associate Professor and Investigator
Stanford University School of Medicine/HHMI
Stanford, CA

Michael G. Kurilla, M.D., Ph.D.
Research Scientist
DuPont Experimental Station
Wilmington, DE

Andrew Lassar, Ph.D.
Associate Professor
Harvard Medical School
Boston, MA

Ethan A. Lerner, M.D., Ph.D.
Associate Professor
Massachusetts General Hospital
Boston, MA

Ellen Li, M.D., Ph.D.
Professor
Washington University School of Medicine
St. Louis, MO

Joachim J. Li, M.D., Ph.D.
Associate Professor
University of California, San Francisco
San Francisco, CA

Michael R. Lieber, M.D., Ph.D.
Professor
University of Southern California School of Medicine
Los Angeles, CA

Daniel V. Madison, Ph.D.
Associate Professor
Stanford University School of Medicine
Stanford, CA

Benjamin L. Margolis, M.D.
Professor and Investigator
University of Michigan/HHMI
Ann Arbor, MI

Michael McClelland, Ph.D.
Director of Molecular Biology
Sidney Kimmel Cancer Center
San Diego, CA

Markus Meister, Ph.D.
Professor
Harvard University
Cambridge, MA

Jonathan Samuel Minden, Ph.D.
Associate Professor
Carnegie Mellon University
Pittsburgh, PA

Denise J. Montell, Ph.D.
Professor
Johns Hopkins University
Baltimore, MD

Andrew Wood Murray, Ph.D.
Professor
Univeristy of California, San Francisco
San Francisco, CA

Timothy F. Osborne, Ph.D.
Associate Professor
University of California, Irvine
Irvine, CA

Michael J. Palazzolo, M.D., Ph.D.
Director of Biosciences
Amgen
Thousand Oaks, CA

Norbert Perrimon, Ph.D.
Professor and Investigator
Harvard Medical School/HHMI
Boston, MA

William A. Petri, Jr., M.D., Ph.D.
Professor
University of Virginia
Charlottesville, VA

Robin E. Reed, Ph.D.
Professor
Harvard Medical School
Boston, MA

Sharon L. Reed, M.D.
Associate Professor
University of California, San Diego
San Diego, CA

Marc L. Reitman, M.D., Ph.D.
Chief, Diabetes Branch, NIDDK
National Institutes of Health
Bethesda, MD

David A. Relman, M.D.
Associate Professor
Stanford University School of Medicine
Stanford, CA

Christopher Mark Rembold, M.D.
Associate Professor
University of Virginia School of Medicine
Charlottesville, VA

Gregory S. Retzinger, M.D., Ph.D.
Associate Professor
University of Cincinnati
Cincinnati, OH

Donald C. Rio, Ph.D.
Professor
University of California, Berkeley
Berkeley, CA

James T. Roberts, M.D., Ph.D.
Member and Investigator
Fred Hutchinson Cancer Research Center/HHMI
Seattle, WA

Shimon Sakaguchi, M.D., Ph.D.
Professor
Kyoto University
Kyoto, Japan

David A. Scheinberg, M.D., Ph.D.
Member
Memorial Sloan-Kettering Cancer Center
New York, NY

Sandra L. Schmid, Ph.D.
Professor
The Scripps Research Institute
La Jolla, CA

David C. Schwartz, Ph.D.
Professor
University of Wisconsin
Madison, WI

Gregg L. Semeza, M.D., Ph.D.
Professor
Johns Hopkins University
Baltimore, MD

Arlene Sharpe, M.D., Ph.D.
Associate Professor
Brigham and Woman's Hospital
Boston, MA

Bradley T. Sheares, Ph.D.
Vice President
Merck & Company, Inc.
West Point, PA

Michael A. Simon, Ph.D.
Associate Professor
Stanford University
Stanford, CA

Peter K. Sorger, Ph.D.
Professor
Massachusetts Institute of Technology
Cambridge, MA

Eric Jay Sorscher, M.D.
Professor
University of Alabama, Birmingham
Birmingham, AL

Ann Stock, Ph.D.
Professor and Investigator
University of Medicine and Dentistry of New Jersey/HHMI
Piscataway, NJ

Robert I. Tepper, M.D.
President
Millennium Pharmaceuticals, Inc.
Cambridge, MA

Marc Tessier-Lavigne, Ph.D.
Professor and Investigator
Stanford University/HHMI
Stanford, CA

Richard A. Van Etten, M.D., Ph.D.
Associate Professor
Harvard Medical School
Boston, MA

Steven A. Wasserman, Ph.D.
Professor
University of California, San Diego
San Diego, CA

M. Gerard Waters, Ph.D.
Director of Laboratory
Merck & Company, Inc.
West Point, PA

Janis J. Weis, Ph.D.
Associate Professor
University of Utah
Salt Lake City, UT

Jeffrey N. Weiser, M.D.
Associate Professor
University of Pennsylvania
Philadelphia, PA

Malcolm R. Whitman, Ph.D.
Associate Professor
Harvard Medical School
Boston, MA

Sandra L. Wolin, M.D., Ph.D.
Associate Professor and Assistant In
Yale University School of Medicine/HHMI
New Haven, CT

Jon P. Woods, M.D., Ph.D.
Associate Professor
University of Wisconsin Medical School
Madison, WI

George D. Yancopoulos, M.D., Ph.D.
President
Regeneron Pharmaceuticals, Inc.
Tarrytown, NY

Martin L. Yarmush, M.D., Ph.D.
Helen A. Benedict Professor
Harvard Medical School
Boston, MA

Tim J. Yen, Ph.D.
Member
Fox Chase Cancer Center
Philadelphia, PA

John Ding-E Young, M.D., Ph.D.
President
The Interplast Group
Livingston, NJ

Appendix E

United Kingdom and Australian Visiting Fellows

Richard J. Benjamin, Ph.D.
Chief Medical Officer
New England Region
American Red Cross
Boston, MA

Claire Henchcliffe, Ph.D.
Director
Parkinson's Institute at New York Hospital
Cornell Medical Center
New York, NY

Ian J. Holt, Ph.D.
Mitochondrial Diseases Group Leader
MRC-Dunn Human Nutrition Unit
Wellcome Trust-MRC Building
Cambridge, United Kingdom

Clare M. Huxley, Ph.D.
Division of Biomedical Sciences Medicine
Imperial College of Science Technology and Medicine
London, United Kingdom

Jordan Raff, Ph.D.
Department of Genetics
Wellcome/CRC Institute
Cambridge, United Kingdom

Guy P. Vigers, Ph.D.
Array BioPharma
Boulder, CO

Charles ffrench-Constant, Ph.D.
Department of Pathology
Wellcome/CRC Institute
Cambridge, United Kingdom

Kenneth Ramsey Howard, Ph.D.
MRC-LMCB
University College
London, United Kingdom

Stephen Philip Jackson, Ph.D.
Professor
Wellcome/CRC Institute
Cambridge, United Kingdom

Richard J. Epstein, Ph.D.
Senior Lecturer
Department of Metabolic Medicine
Imperial College School of Medicine
London, United Kingdom

Simon M. Hughes, Ph.D.
MRC Scientist
MRC Muscle and Cell Motility Unit and Developmental Biology Research
    Centre
The Randall Institute, King's College London
London, United Kingdom

Anthony Hyman, Ph.D.
Max Planck Institute of Molecular CBG
Dresden, Germany

Richard M Durbin, Ph.D.
Head of Informatics Division
Department of Informatics
Wellcome Trust Genome Campus
Cambridge, United Kingdom

Nigel T. Maidment, Ph.D.
Associate Professor
Department of Psychiatry and Behavioral Science
University of California, Los Angeles
Los Angeles, CA

Laurence E. Reid, Ph.D.
Millennium Pharmaceuticals
Cambridge, MA

Mark Rolfe, Ph.D.
Director
Mitotix, Inc.
Cambridge, MA

Alexander R. Duncan, Ph.D.
Cambridge Antibody Technology, Ltd.
Cambridgeshire, United Kingdom

Elizabeth Macintyre-Davi, Ph.D.
Chef de Service
Hematologie Biologique
Hopital Necker-Enfants Malades
Paris, France

Simon James Foote, Ph.D.
Co-Director
Australian Genome Research Facility, Genetics and Bioinformatics Group
The Walter and Eliza Hall Institute of Medical Research
Melbourne, Victoria, Australia

Michelle D. Garrett, Ph.D.
Team Leader
Cancer Research UK Centre for Cancer Therapeutics
at the Institute of Cancer Research
15 Cotswold Road, Sutton, United Kingdom

Kevin Hardwick, Ph.D.
Research Group Leader
Institute of Cell and Molecular Biology
University of Edinburgh
Edinburgh, United Kingdom

Peter Leedman, Ph.D.
Senior Lecturer in Medicine
Lab for Cancer Medicine, WAIM
University of Western Australia
Perth, Western Australia, Australia

Michael G. McHeyzer-Williams, Ph.D.
Associate Professor
Department of Immunology
Scripps Research Institute
La Jolla, CA

Jonathan Millar, Ph.D.
Division of Yeast Genetics
National Institute for Medical Research
London, United Kingdom

Andrew Charles Perkins, Ph.D.
Group Leader, Haematopoiesis
Institute for Molecular Bioscience
University of Queensland
Brisbane, Queensland, Australia

Linda Jane Richards, Ph.D.
Associate Professor
Department of Anatomy and Neurobiology
University of Maryland, Baltimore School of Medicine
Baltimore, MD

Ann Marie Turnley, Ph.D.
Centre for Neuroscience
The University of Melbourne
Melbourne, Victoria, Australia

David L. Vaux, Ph.D.
Cell Death Laboratory
The Walter and Eliza Hall Institute of Medical Research
Melbourne, Victoria, Australia

John Gubbay, Ph.D.
Royal Free Hospital and School of Medicine
London, United Kingdom

Paul Michael Waring, Ph.D.
Department of Pathology
University of Melbourne
Melbourne, Victoria, Australia

Katherine Watson, Ph.D.
(nee Katherine Ann Kelly)
Riddell's Creek, Victoria, Australia

Anamitra Bhattacharyya, Ph.D.
Group Leader for Genome Analysis
Integrated Genomics, Inc.
Chicago, IL

Andrew Chisholm, Ph.D.
Associate Professor
Department of Molecular, Cellular and Developmental Biology
University of California
Santa Cruz, CA

Douglas J. Hilton, Ph.D.
Senior Research Fellow
Cancer Research Unit
The Walter and Eliza Hall Institute of Medical Research
Melbourne, Victoria, Australia

Neil McDonald, Ph.D.
Structural Biology Laboratory
London Research Institute
London, United Kingdom

Andrew David Randall, Ph.D.
Neurology CEDD
GlaxoSmithKline
Essex, United Kingdom

Appendix F

Interview Guides

INTERVIEW GUIDE FOR MARKEY SCHOLARS

I. **Items for all Scholars**

1. What was your reaction when you found out that you had been nominated for and received the Markey Award?

2. Describe how the Markey award affected your independence as a postdoc.
   Were you able to develop your own pilot data?
   Were you able to conduct your own research projects, or were you able to engage in early grant writing?

3. How did the Markey award affect your plans when you were a postdoc?
   Did it make your life more flexible?
   In what ways did it make your life more flexible?
   Did the Markey Award provide you with opportunities other postdocs missed?
   What were those opportunities?
   Describe how receiving the award impacted your postdoc and the relationships you had with colleagues and supervisors.

4. What factors influenced your choice of the first position out of the postdoc?
    Please describe the job search experience.

5. What were your department's expectations of you as a junior faculty member compared with faculty who did not have the immediate support provided by the Markey Award?
    Did the Markey Award have a positive or neutral effect on being hired?
    Did the department reduce the amount of support it provided because of the Markey Award?
    How did this support affect the collegial atmosphere?
    What were your own expectations as a junior faculty member?
    Describe the process that led you to enter the industrial sector.

6. Describe the influence of the Markey Award on funding opportunities.
    What was the prestige/PR value of the Markey award for you?
    Was the Markey Award a help or hindrance in getting additional funding?

7. What sort of teaching responsibilities were expected of you at your first position?
    How have these changed over time?
    What sort of mentoring responsibilities were expected of you in your lab?

8. How did you develop your lab in terms of personnel?
    • how many postdocs have you trained?
    • how many grad students?
    • tell me about the successful ones, the less successful ones.

9. How did the Markey award affect your networking capabilities?
    Was it a help or hindrance in forming bonds with fellow junior faculty?

10. Please describe your current interests in biomedical research.

11. Are you practicing translational research—that is, research that—engaged in clinical trials, or research in human genetics? [If yes] Does your research require IRB approval?

12. Is what you are doing now, what you envisioned yourself doing when you were a Scholar?
    If not, what did you envision yourself doing?
    What factors and situations led you to your current situation?
    In what directions do you see the biomedical enterprise heading and the consequences for your career plans?
    [Ask of those not employed in industry] What types of relationships have you established with the biomedical/ pharmaceutical industry?

II. Item Added for Scholars Who Are M.D.s or M.D./Ph.D.s

13. Do you currently or have you ever practiced medicine?
    [If never practiced] Why did you never practice medicine?
    [If ever practiced] How has your research activity influenced the way you practice(d) medicine?

INTERVIEW GUIDE FOR COMPARISON GROUP MEMBERS

I. Items for all Comparison Group Members

1. How much independence did you have with your research as a postdoctoral fellow? As a junior faculty member?

2. Discuss your ability to set up a lab as a junior faculty member. What about interrelationships with senior faculty, do you think that you were too independent or not independent enough, or were the relationship about right? What impact do you think this level of independence had on your career and scientific achievements?

3. Describe your job search at the end of your postdoctoral fellowship.

4. What things affected your early career as a faculty member and your relationships with other junior faculty in your department?

5. Did your postdoctoral education provide you any opportunities for career flexibility, a change in career direction, or career development/ enhancement? Describe these opportunities.

6. How did your postdoctoral experience affect your visibility within your institution(s)? Did you ever feel that too much was expected of you because of postdocs?

7. How did your postdoctoral education affect your professional network? Affect your visibility within your field?

8. Discuss how changes to your professional network have enhanced your research? How has your research enhanced your networks?

9. Discuss you ability to attract funding from extramural sources. From intramural sources. What factors have affected your ability to obtain funding?

10. Describe how your postdoctoral education affected your ability to attract students, postdoctoral fellows, or other faculty to your lab and/or department.

11. Describe the new scientific ideas, patents, discoveries, licenses, inventions or procedures that developed as a direct or indirect result of your postdoctoral education.

12. Is there anything else you would like to add about your postdoctoral education in general and its impact on your education and career?

II. Items Added for Comparison Group Members Who Are Physicians

13. Do you currently or have you ever practiced medicine?
[If never practiced] Why did you never practice medicine?
[If ever practiced] How has your research activity influenced the way you practice(d) medicine?

INTERVIEW GUIDE FOR MARKEY VISITING FELLOWS

I. Items for all Fellows

1. What was your reaction when you found out that you had been nominated for and received the Markey Visiting Fellows Award?

2. Describe how the Markey award affected your independence as a postdoc. [Were you able to develop your own pilot data, were you able to conduct your own research projects?]

3. How did the Markey award affect your plans following completion of the fellowship? Did it make your life more "flexible"? [In what ways?] Did the Markey Award provide you with opportunities other fellows/postdocs may have missed?

4. Describe the influence of the Markey Award on obtaining subsequent postdoctoral positions. What was the prestige/PR value of the Markey award for you?

5. What was different about postdoctoral research in the United States compared to postdoctoral research in the United Kingdom?

6. What factors influenced your choice of the first position out of the postdoc? Please describe the job search experience.

7. Why did you decide to remain in the United States following the completion of the Markey Fellowship? Why did you decide not to remain in the United States following the completion of the Markey Fellowship?

8. What was the impact of the Markey Fellowship on your research?

9. Please describe your current interests in biomedical research.

10. Are you practicing translational research — that is, research that is engaged in clinical trials, or research in human genetics?

11. Is what you are doing now, what you envisioned yourself doing when you were a Markey Fellow? If not, what did you envision yourself doing? What factors and situations led you to your current situation? In what directions do you see the biomedical enterprise heading and the consequences for your career plans? [Ask of those not employed in industry] What types of relationships have you established with the biomedical/ pharmaceutical industry?

II. Item to Be Added for Fellows Who Are M.D.s or M.D./Ph.D.s

1. Do you currently or have you ever practiced medicine. [If never practiced] Why did you never practice medicine? [If ever practiced] How has your research activity influenced the way you practice(d) medicine?